purposeful
breathing

Meet Dr Greg Smith

For over 30 years I have been a psychologist helping people experiencing difficulties with anxiety, depression, stress management and anger, among other things. The more time has gone on, the more I have refined some simple skills for helping a range of difficulties. Central in this has been the use of conscious breathing. I also work as a lecturer in counselling and psychotherapy and have taught these skills over several years to the graduate students.

My other path to these ideas comes from a lifelong love of yoga. A central part of yoga is *pranayama*, the art and science of breathing. This has been developed and refined over literally thousands of years. In recent years I have studied the exciting developments through which Western science is beginning to provide explanations for many of the things known experientially in the East for so long.

My 'doctor' title comes from a doctorate studying 'Inspiration in Everyday Life'. 'Inspiration' has the dual meaning of both 'being uplifted and infused with an exalted idea or purpose', and also to 'breathe in', so the doctorate allowed me to explore both meanings and their connection.

purposeful breathing

RESET YOUR MIND
IMPROVE YOUR ENERGY
ENHANCE YOUR HEALTH

DR GREG SMITH

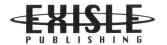

EXISLE
PUBLISHING

First published 2020

Exisle Publishing Pty Ltd
PO Box 864, Chatswood, NSW 2057, Australia
226 High Street, Dunedin, 9016, New Zealand
www.exislepublishing.com

A CiP record for this book is available from the National Library of Australia.

ISBN 978-1-925820-59-1

Designed by Mark Thacker
Typeset in 10.75 on 14.5pt Minion Pro
Printed in China

This book uses paper sourced under ISO 14001 guidelines from well-managed
forests and other controlled sources.

10 9 8 7 6 5 4 3 2 1

Disclaimer
This book is a general guide only and should never be a substitute for the
skill, knowledge and experience of a qualified medical professional dealing
with the facts, circumstances and symptoms of a particular case. The health
information presented in this book is based on the research, training and
professional experience of the author, and is true and complete to the best of
their knowledge. However, this book is intended only as an informative guide;
it is not intended to replace or countermand the advice given by the reader's
personal physician. Because each person and situation is unique, the author and
the publisher urge the reader to check with a qualified healthcare professional
before using any procedure where there is a question as to its appropriateness.
The author, publisher and their distributors are not responsible for any adverse
effects or consequences resulting from the use of the information in this book.
It is the responsibility of the reader to consult a physician or other qualified
healthcare professional regarding their personal care. The intent of the
information provided is to be helpful; however, there is no guarantee of results
associated with the information provided.

For Jane, always beautiful and
brimming with the energy of life.
And for Saxon and Levi, endless
sources of inspiration.

CONTENTS

PART 1

Background information

INTRODUCTION: THE BREATH AS MIND-BODY LINK

I remember as a boy being curious about breathing.

I was a keen sportsman and I can particularly recall a time at football training, running hard and straining for breath. When the time came for a break, I approached the coach and asked him what the best way to breathe was. He looked a little puzzled and said something like 'Just focus on the ball, son.'

To some extent he was right, because different styles of breathing can happen automatically, but when I was painfully struggling for breath I knew there must be more to it.

My interest in breathing has continued over many years.

As a psychologist, I would often notice how people in different emotional states, such as when feeling anxious or depressed, would breathe in quite different ways. Some people would breathe in shallow, rapid patterns. At times people would stop breathing when they were thinking of something upsetting. Often, the most important moments in a therapy session were those moments when a person made an 'emotional shift' and they would begin to breathe more deeply or let out a long sigh of release.

I have also practised yoga for many years and breathing is central to the practice. Yoga promotes a depth of breathing that allows deep relaxation. In yoga the breath is taken to reflect a person's state of mind. Shallow, uneven breathing reflects an agitated mind and slow, deep breathing reflects a calm mind. Yoga also uses the breath to build energy, with *pranayama* being both a control of the breath and a science of energy expansion. In its practices of meditation, yoga builds an awareness of different states of mind and the breath can be used as a tool to change between these states of mind.

The chapters in this book draw upon my experience as a therapist and yoga teacher to explore the ways the breath can be used as a mind–body link. The book outlines a number of simple practices which can be helpful for a range of purposes in everyday life, from managing stress, promoting health and healing, enhancing performance in different areas, or inviting a sense of inspiration.

How to use this book

The breath forms an incredibly powerful mind–body connection. Even though we all breathe all the time, we don't usually pay it much attention.

This book is a manual for simple breathing skills that can rapidly reduce states you don't want (such as stress, anxiety, agitation, depression) and increase states you do want (feeling calmer, stronger, more energized or inspired). These skills are linked with new discoveries from psychology and neuroscience.

For anyone suffering from anxiety, feeling calmer can happen in a breath or two. For anyone wanting to boost performance, the skills in this book will help to get you in 'the zone' of peak performance. As well as the rapid skills, the book also teaches breathing skills for longer term health and healing.

As you read through the book, you'll see various breathing styles, or exercises, scattered throughout the chapters. Some exercises (such as the standing breathing styles on pp. 164–70) can be done in a sequence if preferred, so they appear together. There is also an appendix on p. 186 that lists each breathing style featured in the book.

I have included numerous case studies to show you how I have used different breathing styles to help clients. The case studies are based on real clients but their names and identifying details have changed. Some cases are composites of typical features of many clients.

Breathing skills are a treasure.

Control the breath and you control the mind.
—Buddhist saying

State of breathing reflects state of mind.
—Yoga saying

1

BREATHING AS A MASTER SWITCH

The breath is a remarkably powerful mind–body connection.

Although we all breathe everyday it remains a largely unconscious process. This means our breathing often changes in important ways without us being aware of it. Anxiety, anger, deep calm or steady concentration each have their own patterns of breathing and we move between different styles of breathing every day without usually realizing it. If we can recognize these styles of breathing, we can also consciously change them and this in turn produces a change in our emotional state. We can therefore use changes to a pattern of breathing to change our mood and mental states.

For example, if you are anxious, the breath is often shallow and sharp, and changing your breathing to slow and deep, using the diaphragm, will lower your level of anxiety. This change is not usually so powerful as to make you totally relaxed in a few moments, but it is usually enough to 'take the edge off' the anxiety and 'crank it down a few notches'. For someone suffering anxiety this is usually enough to allow them to think more clearly about the situation and decide upon what additional strategies to use to help.

In my work as a psychologist I have taught simple 'belly breathing' or diaphragmatic breathing to literally hundreds of people with severe anxiety, and they learn how to rapidly calm themselves. Severe anxiety can be very debilitating, and if someone was offered a pill that could reduce their anxiety levels by 30 per cent in one or two minutes, there would be a big market for the medication. The same thing, however, can be done with simple breathing, and anxiety is just one application. Breathing skills can be used to change states of mind, concentrate better, enhance performance and much more.

Everyday styles of breathing

The following are typical styles of breathing linked with different moods or emotional states. I notice them for myself, as my own breathing changes with different emotions, but more particularly see them over and again in people who come to see me for assistance in therapy.

Each of these breaths is typical, and the style of breathing may of course change from person to person. They are not recommended styles of breathing, but highlight how breathing changes with mood. If you try each style of breathing you can see how much it might relate to your own breathing patterns as they link with your own emotional changes.

If you would like to try each of these breaths for a few rounds, do it gently. For all of the breathwork in the book, check with your doctor if you have any concerns.

You might like to just read these descriptions, but if you try them, be aware that the effect is often subtle and is also impacted by perhaps feeling a little self-conscious doing something new and different. Sometimes people feel nothing much and then do it more and more, and then all of a sudden go 'whoa' as it crosses a threshold of awareness. So go slowly and stop if you feel any discomfort.

Anxious breathing

Generally, people who are anxious tend to breathe high into the top of the chest and hold the breath in. The breath leaks out a little slowly over several seconds, rather than being strongly exhaled, and then there is another breath high in the chest. The in-breath often has a gasping quality to it.

The pattern is: inhale high, hold, hardly exhale at all, inhale high again.

If you do several rounds of this you are likely to find you produce a state of being tense and on edge that would usually physically correlate with anxiety.

Panic breathing

Panic is often accompanied by hyperventilation, whereby people breathe in and out very fast into the upper chest. It is quick and shallow. Generally, when people breathe this way they tend to 'spin out'. The oxygen and carbon dioxide exchange gets distorted and the old-fashioned remedy of breathing into a paper bag is one method people use to rebalance this.

You probably don't need to try this breath to imagine it, but if you do try it, do so carefully and stop if you start to feel the sensation of 'spinning out' that it can induce.

Chronic hyperventilation

For many people, a mild version of panic breathing can become chronic. They breathe fast and shallow as a normal pattern. This can have a huge impact on their body chemistry and be linked with a range of medical conditions. For these people, learning to breathe slowly and deeply can be life-changing. Read more about chronic hyperventilation in Chapter 4.

Stress breath

Many people, if very stressed or threatened, close down their breathing to a minimal level, with hardly any movement of their chest or belly at all. It can feel almost as if there is some animal response of 'playing possum', as if a predator was nearby and the body is attempting to stop all movement, even the movement of the breath. For some people who experience stress, this becomes their predominant breathing pattern.

Blocking emotion

Often when people experience powerful or unpleasant emotions, they hold their breath as if they are bracing themselves. I remember seeing *Alien* years ago. As the film moved into a particularly suspenseful scene, where it appeared the alien might jump out, I remember the sharp intake of breath from seemingly the entire movie theatre. This would be held silently for a few moments until the suspense was broken, and there were little shrieks and then a ripple of nervous laughter.

People living in chronically stressful situations can develop this kind of breath-holding, which inadvertently keeps them on edge.

Some of the ways we block our breathing can become habitual, and opening beyond them can feel liberating. In therapy, or in other forms of self-development such as yoga, people often find that as they extend the breath it releases some memories from a time when the breath was initially blocked. Done in a controlled way, this can be a helpful release.

Depressed breathing

People who are deeply saddened or depressed can appear to exhale more than they inhale. I often see people breathing out in the manner of a deep sigh, then the breath is held out for some moments before there is a short breath in and another sighing exhale. This breath is usually deeper in the lower chest, in contrast to the anxious breath, which is often high in the chest.

Having longer exhalations than inhalations tends to lower the body's energy, and holding the breath out tends to lower it even more.

If you would like to try this for a few moments, you will find it tends to produce a state of feeling de-energized and physically flat, as if tired. These traits physically correlate with depression. Of course, you won't usually want to make yourself depressed, so it may be enough just to read about it.

Although it is an exaggeration, generally people who are anxious don't breathe out and people who are depressed don't breathe in.

Enraged breathing

People who are enraged tend to breathe into the front of the chest, pumping the solar plexus area just below the sternum. When I think of this, I often have an image of the New Zealand All Blacks rugby team doing a *haka* before the start of an international match, both pumping themselves up and projecting a message of intimidation to their foes.

It is easy to picture an enraged person, nostrils flaring and chest pumping, charged with energy and ready to attack. Breathing to this central area in the front of the body seems to link with this sense of being pumped up and ready to fight.

Trying this style of breathing while calmly reading this text might not get you enraged but you are likely to feel something of the 'pumped up' feeling and the sense that this may be directed at some outward object. This is in contrast to the 'spinning out' of fast, high panic breathing, and also contrasts with strong, fast breathing to the belly, which charges the body but also allows a more controlled, centred feeling.

Habitual breathing

For the most part breathing goes on unconsciously, unless we stop and deliberately control it. But breathing patterns are continually changing in line with our interactions. If we are shocked we tend to gasp, if we are sad we often sigh; our breathing rate speeds up or slows down depending on our level of excitation or calm. There is a range of ways in which these bodily responses link with our experience of the world.

Breathing patterns may reflect long-term embodied patterns of responding, as well as immediate responses. If you suffer from chronic anxiety you may have a pattern of breathing into the upper chest and holding your breath, or you might overbreathe in a low-level, ongoing hyperventilation. Such patterns can become habitual, rather than just lasting for a few anxious moments.

Attention to the breath has long been important in Eastern traditions such as yoga. Smooth, slow breathing is more inducive and reflective of a state of calmness, as opposed to sharp or fast breathing. When inhalations are longer than the exhalations energy levels rise, and vice versa.

Stress is a significant factor. After being stressed, our bodies can reset in ways that have damaging long-term effects. Some people can become hyper-vigilant and 'on alert' most of the time, with breathing patterns interlinking with their mental and emotional states. Over time, people may suffer from the results of stress in a range of physical ways.

All of us will have habitual patterns of breathing which influence mood for better or for worse, but the good news is that changing styles of breathing can have a profound influence on mood and health.

Breathing as therapy

When people become 'stuck' in psychological difficulties, such as depression, anxiety or chronic post-traumatic stress, they are usually also stuck in habitual and limited breathing patterns. The case studies below show how I've worked with some clients to help them move from habitual breathing patterns to more helpful breathing styles.

Nick

Nick came to see me for help with his anxiety. He described being anxious a lot of the time, especially in social situations. He had Asperger's syndrome, which meant that he had difficulty reading other people's social cues, and this in turn fed his social anxiety. As we talked about this background I noticed his breathing was quite strained.

I asked if he would like ways to calm himself and he was keen to learn some of these techniques. I gave some information about breathing and mood. I asked where he would place his level of anxiety at that moment on a scale of 0 to 10, where 0 was totally relaxed and 10 was extreme anxiety. He said about an 8.

When I asked him to take a deep breath, he breathed in what looked like a gulping action and lifted his shoulders high, breathing into the very top of his chest.

I taught him diaphragmatic breathing, which he did for several breaths. I asked again how he felt and he said he was now a 3 on the scale. He said he felt 'lightheaded in a good way' and 'blissful'. He had never focused on styles of breathing before and the whole thing was a revelation to him. The process, from beginning to talk about breathing to teaching it and practising, only took a few minutes. Nick was very clear that this was a skill he would practise every day.

Vicki

Vicki came into my office beaming. She was clearly excited and said she wanted to shout in celebration when she had gotten into the carpark. Then she told me that she had driven from her home to my office.

About twelve months earlier, Vicki had been in a horrific car accident. While physically only suffering bruising, the accident had a deep psychological impact. She became terrified of travelling in cars as a passenger and could not drive at all. She saw a psychologist, who told her she would never drive again. The accident came after a time of other problems in her life and she became quite withdrawn, ceased working and was spending long periods at home.

Eventually Vicki was referred to me for help with her post-traumatic responses to being in a car. She could manage to go on short trips with her husband driving, but would jump and shout if any car pulled close to them. She avoided other car travel, and would feel sick when she occasionally caught a bus.

When she first came to my office, Vicki was clearly extremely tense. As with many people I see who have post-traumatic stress, her breathing was very high and constrained; shallow to just the top of the chest. I spent time trying to help her breathe more deeply, using the diaphragm and breathing as if into the belly. Initially this was impossible for Vicki. It was as if her diaphragm, her solar plexus, and the area just under her ribs had been frozen. We talked about this, as if her body had become stuck in that moment of shock and fear.

Slowly and gently we worked to help her breathe more deeply and she would practise at home. By the third session she was able to breathe deeply again, and as she did this she was able to begin, bit by bit, to relax. Over time I asked Vicki to sit in her car while it was parked in her driveway, to help her get used to once again being in the car and feeling more in control, using the breathing when needed to calm herself. A few weeks later she drove herself to the appointment.

More than this, other emotions that had been blocked when Vicki was frozen in fear, could now surface. She began expressing more excitement, joy, happiness, indignation and sadness as she again responded more freely to what was happening in her daily life and what had happened over the last couple of years. Vicki still faced many challenges, but freeing up her breathing had been a key to unlocking potentials for further recovery.

Jenny

Jenny came to see me describing problems with controlling her emotions. She had ongoing sadness, and would often break down in tears. Her doctor had prescribed an antidepressant, which she had been taking for the last five months.

Her problems with sadness and depression had begun two years earlier when her relationship of seven years ended. The relationship had been deteriorating but it was her boyfriend who broke it off. She said she was upset and just put up with her sadness for several months, but when it continued for more than a year she felt it wasn't right, and eventually after about eighteen months saw her doctor.

She felt the medication had helped a little but sought psychological assistance to get over the sadness and to have control over her tearfulness. On broader discussion, Jenny said she felt often disappointed that at 29 she had not achieved much in life. She worked part-time as a retail assistant, but was now also in her second year of university studies.

In the session we identified longer and shorter-term goals. Her immediate goal was to feel 'lighter' as she felt so heavy most of the time. We discussed breathing as one immediate option for helping to feel lighter.

In looking at her breath it seemed very constricted — it was hard to see anything happen, any movement of chest or belly. When asked to take a deep breath, she breathed quite high in her chest, as most adults do. We then progressed to teach belly breathing, both slow and in a stronger muscular fashion.

I described the *hara* point (below and behind the navel; see p. 104) and how to breathe to this point.

After that we progressed to full breathing, beginning in the belly and progressing up to the middle and upper chest and then out from upper, middle and lower. After doing some rounds of this we then tried to direct the full breath more to the back of the body, and did several rounds of this breathing.

After this, I asked how Jenny felt. She said enthusiastically 'Much lighter', and smiled, clearly happy with the difference.

Jenny seemed keen to practise the breathing techniques and said she would practise for 20 minutes a day. I told her 20 minutes was great, but even a few minutes a few times a day would be very good.

I went through how to use the different breaths: slow diaphragmatic breathing to calm anxiety; muscular, strong, breathing if feeling fragile and wanting to feel strong; slow, full, back breath for a calm and more meditative state; a full, strong, medium-paced back breath for energy and focus; full frontal breathing only if she felt she wanted to release some emotion.

Jenny said that when doing the breathing she became aware of what felt like a blockage releasing in her solar plexus area — she said 'here' and placed her hand in the centre of her upper abdomen just below the rib cage. She said she felt like she hadn't previously been breathing below that point, and as if something had been stuck there. I discussed with her that often people going through times of difficult emotion will block and hold tension there.

As she felt calmer and stronger, Jenny was much better placed to talk though other issues, including working through unresolved grief following her break-up.

A very restricted range of breath limits your emotional responses. This emotional restriction may be helpful in the short term — such as staying alert to threat or not wanting to break down and sob in public — and may be initially conscious or unconscious. But in the longer term it can become 'stuck' and very unhelpful. Changing the breathing can open up more emotional freedom.

Changing modes

In the play *The Bourgeois Gentleman* by Molière, Monsieur Jourdain asks his philosophy teacher to help him compose a love letter. The teacher asks if he should write it in poetry or prose. Monsieur Jourdain does not want poetry and has to ask what prose is. When told that prose is what he speaks all the time, he is delighted to discover he is a master of such a skill. All the while, he has been an expert in prose without even realizing it!

Like Monsieur Jourdain, all of us are masters of many skills which go unrecognized in day-to-day life. One of these skills is the way we 'change modes'.

While people sometimes talk about being in 'work mode' or 'party mode', we change 'modes' throughout the day, without usually being aware of them. Stress, depression, creative states, 'survival mode' and the 'zone' of peak performance might all be seen as particular modes.

Often we get stuck in a particular mode without realizing it. Staying too long in any one mode is a sure way to induce stress, frustration and a vague sense of being a robot.

In any mode, ways of thinking, acting, feeling and relating are interlinked. For example, if someone is depressed, they tend to feel depressed, think depressing thoughts, notice all the negative things around them (but not the positive things) and often avoid other people. If someone is in the 'zone' of peak performance, they tend to be fully absorbed in the task, active, energized and calmly focused.

While such modes happen every day, the idea of modes is radical. It goes against many deep-rooted convictions in Western thought, such as those which hold the mind to be separate from the body and reason to be separate from emotion. Although the 'mind/body split' has become an outdated concept in recent medical advances, it is still a dichotomy that remains pervasive in both healthcare and broader Western culture, and acts to obscure the ways that thinking involves a body which is actively responding, feeling and perceiving. Thoughts, emotions and perceptions are not separate objects in everyday life but occur as intertwined aspects of living in the world.

Each mode offers different types of awareness and different ways of knowing and acting. They reflect the way that mind, body, emotion and language are intertwined as aspects of the one living process.

The breath is also linked to these modes. Different modes are linked to different breathing patterns. Changing breathing patterns can allow us to enter different modes. In particular, if you are stuck in a mode you don't like, simple controlled breathing allows a way to step out of it and refocus.

On subtle levels we shift modes dozens of times each day. Stress, anger, depression, play and inspiration might all be seen as particular states of mind, with different physical and emotional orientations.

A clear example is the particular mode related to the 'fight or flight' response, a natural response that occurs in humans and animals when faced with danger. This is useful in an evolutionary sense, as the release of adrenaline and other physical changes help in either running away faster or fighting better. The brain also goes into something of a short circuit, so that we can notice and respond to danger well, but are not very creative or clear-thinking. This mode and all its associated changes are a great help if you are about to be hit by a truck, but not so helpful if you are about to give a talk to your work colleagues.

Some modes might be highly desirable. Others, like stress, can be harmful if we get stuck in it for too long. Even someone who is perpetually cheerful can become grating on their companions if cheerful is the only mode they have, and they can be limited in their response to serious issues. The important point here is to notice the ways we move in and out of different modes. Once we recognize these modes we can recognize unhelpful

ones and consciously choose to change them. Sometimes it may be changing the degree — you might not be able to stop being depressed just by
choosing it, but you can have more power in being able to lessen its severity
and more choice in how to respond to it. The more awareness you have of
these modes, the more choice you have over moving between them.

There are many techniques to help change our mind–body states.
Breathing skills are especially easy and effective. Breathing can be used as
the 'reset' switch to change modes.

Sometimes our pattern of breathing is part of a particular mode, and at
times it can also trigger particular reactions.

Max

Max had a phobia about public speaking. While a very confident young
man in most areas of his life, speaking in front of group triggered a
sense of panic. It had begun in high school after a bad experience
presenting to a class and was severe enough that when he went to
university he chose subjects based in part on whether the assessment
involved group presentations — if a subject involved speaking in front
of a group, he chose another subject. He worked on it over time, practising reading aloud and engaging in self-development courses, but the
problem persisted.

When he described this to me in detail, it became clear it was not
really associated with negative thinking but felt like a physical reaction. I had him give a practice presentation to me, reading aloud from a
text. As he did this, I noticed he would read quite long sections of text
then take in a sharp intake of breath. When he read shorter sections of
text (and was not out of breath) he still took in this sharp intake. The
breathing pattern itself was the key trigger of his anxiety — the sharp
intake kicked off the fight or flight response (the sympathetic nervous
system). Such a breathing pattern was unconscious, but once he practised consciously changing it, allowing himself to pause and take a slow
controlled inhale, he overcame the phobia. He went on to enjoy giving
presentations, and now regularly does public speaking.

2

BREATHING AWARENESS

The first step in purposeful breathing is to become more aware of the breath and which parts of the body are involved with different styles of breathing. A simple way to do this is just to take a few breaths with full awareness. Read the section below as a guide, then close your eyes and just let your breathing happen naturally without directing it.

CONSCIOUS BREATHING

Notice which parts of your body move as you breathe in and as you breathe out. Does your upper chest move more or your lower chest? How much does your belly move? How much do your back ribs move? Do the sides of your chest move? Are you breathing through your nose or mouth? If through your nose, is the air flowing more through one nostril than the other? Which parts of the nostril are most touched by the air — is the air drawn more over the lower or upper edges of the nostrils? Notice any other sensations as you breathe.

Rest for a moment and then count your breaths — how many breaths are there in 30 seconds (multiply by two for breaths per minute)?

Then take a fuller breath, deliberately breathing more deeply for a few rounds and notice what happens then, asking all the same questions as above.

Then notice your posture, and how this might affect the breath. If you notice you are leaning forward or back, slumping or leaning in any way, exaggerate that a tiny bit and notice how that feels. Don't judge anything as right or wrong, just notice.

Another way to build awareness is to place one hand on your chest, over your heart, and one hand on your belly, at about the navel. Notice which hand moves more with the inhalation and which hand moves more with the exhalation.

These awareness exercises are good to return to occasionally. You can notice changes in the breath if you are in different emotional states or after you have practised some of the breaths listed in later chapters.

The anatomy of breathing

When you are learning different styles of breathing it is usually best just to try and see how it feels. Thinking about what is working anatomically can feel too technical and be a distraction in the early stages. Once you have tried some different breathing styles, however, some knowledge of the anatomy involved is invaluable.

While breathing is so simple that we do it without thinking, the anatomy of breathing is very complex, and some aspects of the physiology are still not fully understood.

Nonetheless, for breathing awareness there are several key points. The air is taken in through the nose or mouth, then goes through the throat and through branching passages until it reaches the alveoli (the tiny air sacks in which the air and blood exchange oxygen, carbon dioxide and waste gases).

The lungs are a bit pear shaped — there is more of the lungs and more of the alveoli in the lower part. This means breathing deeply rather than high in the chest is a more effective breath.

While the musculature involved in breathing is complex, it can be simplified to three key components: the diaphragm, the muscles of the middle chest (especially the intercostal muscles between the ribs) and the complex collection of muscles around the shoulders linked with the upper chest. This links with three types of breathing: lower, middle and upper.

But the most important muscle involved in breathing is the diaphragm.

The diaphragm

The diaphragm is a dome shaped sheet of muscle that runs across the body under the lungs, roughly level with the bottom of the ribcage. Breathing as if into the belly utilizes the diaphragm, drawing it out and down. You can learn to control the diaphragm directly, using it and strengthening it like any muscle.

Most adults, when asked to take a deep breath, usually breathe quite high in the chest. It is as if we are aware the lungs are in the chest so it seems logical to push the chest out and up in order to take a full breath. By contrast, if you look at young children (two or three year olds) when they are relaxed and lying down, it is their belly that moves with the breath.

Many people use the rib muscles and the upper muscles near the shoulders, but generally, it is far more calming and effective to breathe using the diaphragm as the primary muscle of respiration. While the effects of breathing diaphragmatically have been known for a long time, recent research has found more of the reasons why, especially that breathing diaphragmatically stimulates the vagus nerve (see p. 41), which relaxes the body.

When at rest, the diaphragm is like an umbrella or a parachute that curves up under the ribcage. The resting muscle fibres are longer and the lungs are raised. The strands of the muscles connect to a central tendon, a fibrous tissue called an aponeurosis, which sits along the high point of the dome. This central tendon provides a point of connection for all the diaphragm's

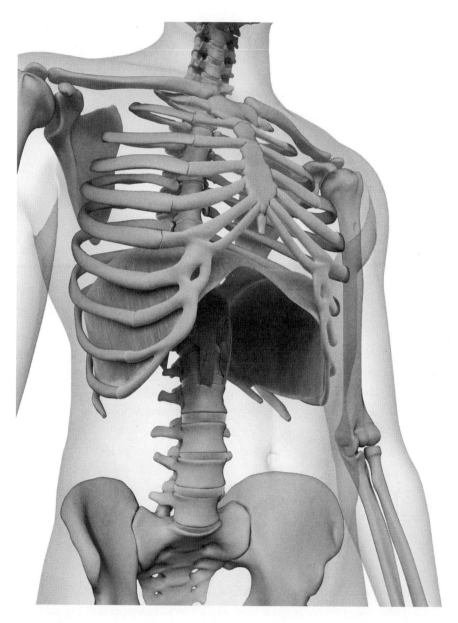

Diaphragm

muscle fibres, which pull against the tendon at one end, with the other end attached to the lower ribs. Think of the bicep: when we curl up our arm and tense the bicep, the muscle fibres contract, becoming shorter and thicker, and the bicep bulges. When the muscle fibres of diaphragm are contracted, they shorten and pull down the central membrane and the entire diaphragm. The diaphragm becomes flatter and thicker, less domed and more like a flat sheet across the bottom of the ribs. This has the effect of pulling down on the lungs and expanding out the lower ribs, creating more space and low pressure in the lungs so air comes in. The pulling down and thickening of the diaphragm muscle fibres also causes the belly to move forward a little, as it pushes down on the organs of the abdomen and the lower ribs to expand. Among other things, diaphragmatic breathing gives a gentle massage of the abdominal organs.

Just to make it a little more complex, all of the muscles involved in breathing can work in different ways depending on which areas we keep fixed and which we allow to move. So if the muscles of the abdomen are held firmly, then the movement of the diaphragm as it contracts will open the ribs and chest more, but usually it is better to allow the gentle movement of the belly.

Not many of us stop to pay much attention to our ribs, so it is worth using your fingers to feel along the bottom edges of the lowest ribs. You can notice that the front ribs are higher, and their line descends downwards as you follow the ribs back. The diaphragm also has more room for movement at the back, as the muscle fibres are longer from the attachment at the back of the ribs to the central tendinous area.

When you breathe diaphragmatically, you can feel the movement by placing your hands on the lowest ribs, feeling them expand on the inhalation. There is more movement at the front, because the back ribs are more restricted by the spine, but ideally the movement is of the front, back and sides gently expanding as you inhale. If you try it, be aware that many people don't breathe this way, so it may take a little practice.

While inhalation entails the active expansion of the lungs, exhalation can be passive as the basic elastic force of the lungs allows the diaphragm to relax back upwards, and the diaphragmatic muscle fibres relax back to a resting state (domed upwards).

Breathing slowly using the diaphragm has a calming and centring effect, and the diaphragmatic breath is a key foundational breath. There are other muscles we can use as well (but more of that later).

The breath itself is very simple, although sometimes it can take a while for people to 'get it' if they have been breathing in other ways. Breathing in, the diaphragm pulls down, thickens and expands out, expanding the lungs and drawing in air; breathing out, it relaxes and lengthens upwards, lower ribs and belly draw in and the lungs contract, as in the illustration.

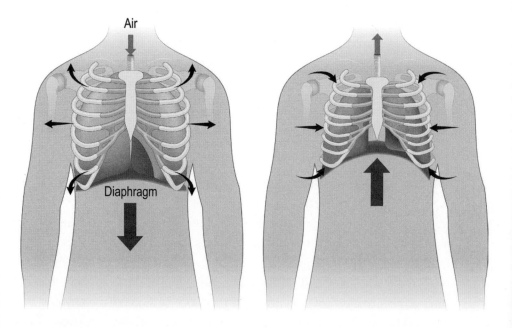

Breathing

The other muscles

The second mechanism involves the muscles of the ribs, the intercostal muscles. These run between each of the ribs in two layers — external and internal intercostals. They are largely responsible for breathing into the mid chest. If the top rib is held fixed, the intercostals draw the ribs together, opening out and lifting up as they do so, opening the chest and lungs to inhale — a bit like pulling up the handle of a bucket. And if the lowest ribs are held fixed the contraction pulls the ribs in and down, leading to an exhalation. Some of the intercostals can be used (such as just the higher or lower ones) rather than all of them at once.

Other muscles of the chest and back are also involved in breathing into the chest, but there is no particular need to identify them here, or to isolate control of them. Generally speaking, we engage them just by thinking about where we want the breath to go.

Muscles used for clavicular breathing

There is a complex range of muscles in the upper chest and around the shoulders which are used when breathing using the very upper chest. This is called clavicular breathing, after the clavicle or collarbone. Engaging this area can be helpful if you are taking a really full breath, adding it to the diaphragmatic and chest movement. In this breath, the shoulders are widened and pulled back a little (rather than lifted) and the upper chest opened. The upper intercostals are involved in clavicular breathing, as are other muscles of the neck, shoulders and upper chest. You can begin to feel the muscles involved by practising taking the breath higher. Importantly, for some people this is their primary (rather than secondary) means of breathing — when asked to take a deep breath, they lift up their shoulders. If this is a consistent style of breathing it places stress on muscles that are only meant to assist breathing (as well as doing other things) and over time tends to be inefficient and exhausting, often leading to neck and shoulder pain.

Specialist breathing muscles

Some additional muscles are used just for inhalation or just for exhalation.

An important set of muscles for exhalation are the abdominals, especially the rectus abdominus, the twin set of muscles that are linked with the 'six-pack' look (the six-pack comes from the muscles being spaced by connections with aponeurotic tendonous areas, like the tendon of the diaphragm). The abdominals connect at one end at the pubic bone and at the other attach to the sternum and costal cartilage of the lower ribs. This muscle, and the muscles on the sides of the abdomen (transverse abdominus and obliques), can extend the exhalation by pulling in, contracting the lower ribs and drawing in the abdominal organs, allowing the diaphragm to rise further and the ribs to draw in, thus expelling more air. This action of extending the exhalation can have may benefits for specific purposes, especially calming (see p. 66).

The pelvic muscles

Finally, there are the muscles at the base of the pelvis which form the pelvic floor. There are superficial and deeper muscles, of which the deeper ones form a diaphragm, or a bowl shape at the base of the pelvis (while allowing the relevant passages through). While obviously removed from the lungs and relatively small, these muscles are important for keeping tone and shape as the abdominal organs move up and down with the breath, and also for extending the exhalation, as they can link with beginning a cascade of movements of exhalation. Good tone in these often-neglected muscles is surprisingly important for all the lower abdominal and pelvic organs. In Eastern terms, good tone prevents energy from 'leaking' out, but our main focus will on using them for a few specific breaths.

We shall come back to using specific muscles, but for now the main focus is the diaphragm, and the awareness that you can breathe lower, higher or more fully using different regions or all of them.

Volumes

All these different muscles and movements means that there is also a huge variation in the amount of breath we can take in.

The average resting breath is generally quite small, about 0.5 litre.

It is a common misconception that the more we breathe the better, but this is no more true than saying that the faster our heart beats the better. We may want our heart rate to be able to go up to 140 beats per minute or more when we are playing sport but no one would want it staying at 140 when in the office. A normal adult resting heart rate is between 60 and 100 beats per minute, and generally a slower the heart rate is an indicator of better health — some athletes may have a resting heart rate as low as 40.

Breathing at rest is similar. For an average healthy male the maximum amount that can be breathed in and out is about 4.5 to 5 litres of air (about a quarter less for females and varying with body size, posture, health, etc.).

Breathing volume

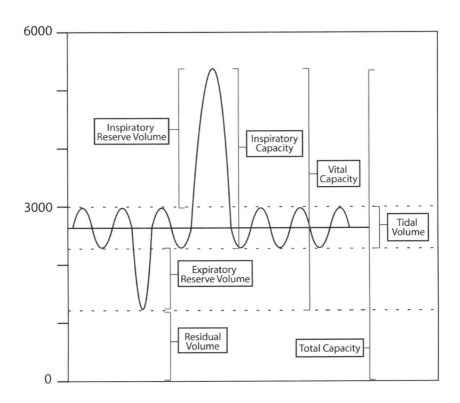

The full volume of the lungs is up to about 6 litres but there is always about a litre or more that can't be exhaled at any one time (due to a limit on how constricted the lungs can be, and so they don't completely collapse).

The best breathing at rest is quite gentle but we have great capacity to inhale or exhale more when it suits us, and doing so will have specific effects that can be used for specific purposes.

The nose knows

If you are exercising vigorously, you may need to breathe through your mouth just to get enough air in and out. In general, however, it is usually better to breathe through your nose. The passages through the nose and sinuses are designed for the breath. They are surprisingly long, have nasal hairs acting as a natural filter, and mucous membranes with which the breath is humidified and brought towards body temperature. Dust and foreign matter is caught and/or filtered.

The nose is not as straightforward as it might at first appear. The obvious part of the nose — that external bit in the middle of your face — is just the beginning of things. Air enters through the nostrils and what is called the *vestibule of the anterior portion of the nose*. A vestibule is an antechamber or lobby, an entrance to something else. Anatomically, it is a chamber or channel leading to another area. Behind this cartilaginous area the nasal septum divides two nasal cavities. At the top of the cavities are the olfactory nerve endings, enabling our sense of smell, and at the back are orifices called the *internal nares* at the top of the *pharynx*. Inside the nasal cavities the walls have many tiny bones called *nasal conchae*, which give the surface many ridges and recesses, and the flow of air is moved around by larger ridges called *turbinates*. The gentle turbulence this creates enhances the process of the air being warmed and humidified. The whole area is lined with mucous membranes which are warm and moist, have many tiny hairs and contain cells that secrete a sticky mucus that includes an antibacterial enzyme. This all acts to pick up any dust particles and prevent bacteria and harmful substances from entering the body.

While these aspects of breathing have been known for a long time, there is, incredibly, new research still emerging about nose breathing. In the 1990s it was discovered that nitric oxide is produced through the paranasal sinuses and acts as an important agent for many body functions, including dilating the blood vessels (more on this in Chapter 3).[1] Breathing through the nose means that the air stimulates the olfactory bulb, central in our sense of smell; and recent discoveries suggest that slow breathing has an effect on the olfactory bulb that goes beyond just smell, to tune the activity of the entire cortex, which is to say it tunes all the higher functions of the brain.[2]

When breathing through the mouth, by contrast, the air goes straight in without the filtering, warming and humidifying that occurs with nose breathing. The mouth is also a much bigger opening, so controlling the flow of air is much less precise — it is easy to dump the air out on the exhale, and easy to overbreathe, which can lead to many problems (see p. 49). If your nose is blocked you can, of course, vary the amount of air going through the mouth by varying the opening, such as imaging you are breathing through a straw. This controls against overbreathing and allows a small warming and humidifying effect as the air flows over the tongue and through the throat.

Breathing through the nose also allows the breath to be more finely regulated. As you practise the breathing styles in this book, you will develop a more finely tuned awareness of when the breath is jerky and uneven, and when it is smooth and regular. Almost everyone begins with an uneven breath, and breathing through the nose allows the development of a greater control and refinement in breathing. Breathing through the nose also regulates the breath better in an easy and natural way.

The importance of breathing through the nose has been central in yoga and many Eastern traditions of health and healing. Yogi Ramacharaka, writing in 1904, saw it is as central to the health or ills of society:

The breathing mechanism of Man [sic] is so constructed that he may breathe either through the mouth or the nasal tubes, but it

is a matter of vital importance to him which method he follows, as one brings health and strength and the other disease and weakness.

... alas! the ignorance among civilized people regarding this simple matter is astounding. We find people in all walks of life habitually breathing through their mouths and allowing their children to follow their horrible and disgusting example.

... No animal, excepting man, sleeps with the mouth open or breathes through the mouth, and in fact it is believed that it is only civilized man who so perverts nature's functions ...[3]

Nothing in this book is quite so dogmatic, and there may be times when you choose to breathe through your mouth, such as in vigorous exercise or controlled exhalations, or for a cooling breath. But for the most part, the nose is designed for breathing. The mouth has other great functions, and if we tried to use the nose for eating or kissing, I doubt it would work very well. Some things are for the mouth and some for the nostrils.

Details of specific styles of breathing are outlined in Chapter 6, but for now just noticing occasionally whether you are breathing high or low, fast or slow, nose or mouth is helpful in developing awareness.

3

KEY MECHANISMS

Why does purposeful breathing work? There are a few key principles that underpin the breathing skills of this book, and which will inform the later information on which breathing styles produce which effects and why.

This chapter gives you a bit of the science behind it, some of which is quite new. Understanding the mechanisms will help inform the practices (but if you don't care about *why* and just want to get to *how*, feel free to skip this chapter).

Oxygen is your best friend

No surprises here. Pretty much everyone will know that we need oxygen to survive. It is the crucial element that we extract from the air we breathe. It is probably the most valuable substance on Earth. After all, no one ever died from a lack of diamonds, and we can survive for a few weeks without food, a few days without water but only a few minutes without oxygen.

Oxygen plays a crucial role in the functioning of all the cells of the body. When we breathe in the air goes through the airway, which branches into smaller and smaller passages (bronchioles) until reaching tiny sacks called alveoli in the lungs. These have thin walls and are surrounded by tiny blood vessels so that gases can be exchanged. Oxygen is taken up by the red blood cells (haemoglobin cells) and carbon dioxide is released back into the alveoli to be exhaled. This oxygen–carbon dioxide exchange happens with every breath, but can be impeded or enhanced as shall be described below. Once taken up by the red blood cells in the lungs, the oxygen is taxied around the bloodstream to be delivered to all the cells of the body, which then use it for energy.

Carbon dioxide is your other best friend

When oxygen reaches our cells it is used in a process called *cellular respiration*, through which energy is created and carbon dioxide (CO_2) is a waste product. The red blood cells that delivered the oxygen pick up the CO_2 and take it back to the lungs for us to get rid of with exhalation.

Most people know of CO_2 as a waste product, and there is a common misconception that we need to get rid of it and the more we get rid of the better. While we need to get rid of an excess of it, carbon dioxide plays many important roles in our body and general health. Of course, if you only breathed carbon dioxide you would drop off the perch quite quickly, but too little CO_2 creates many problems, and it is the balance of oxygen to carbon dioxide that matters.

Oxygen is far less soluble than CO_2. When oxygen enters the body through breathing, a small amount remains dissolved in the blood but over 98 per cent is attached to haemoglobin and carried by the red blood cells. When the oxygen is carried around the body, it is released where it is needed and the red blood cells pick up carbon dioxide. About 20 per cent of the carbon dioxide is carried in this way but CO_2 is also dissolved in the blood, where there is a balance of CO_2 and related chemicals, principally bicarbonate and carbonic acid. The carbon dioxide has a significant role in affecting the acid–alkaline level in the blood (actually, the blood is a little alkaline at a pH of 7.4). The body places a vital priority on keeping the acid–alkaline balance and subtle changes can have noticeable effects (big changes would be deadly). Different rates of breathing mean more CO_2 remains dissolved or is released on the exhalation (as it diffuses through the walls of the alveoli). This affects CO_2 levels in the blood, which in turn has a range of effects.

An important function of CO_2 is that it relaxes the smooth muscles in the walls of major blood vessels — arteries, arterioles and major veins contain smooth muscle within their walls, with less of the muscle as the veins become smaller. This relaxation acts to dilate the blood vessels, so that more CO_2 means the blood vessels open out more and less means they constrict. This has a very efficient effect: when you are using certain muscles they use up more oxygen and release more CO_2, which then means the blood vessels supplying the muscles open more to bring in more blood where it is needed.

As well as this, the body has another neat trick: if there is more CO_2 in a particular area, the oxygen in that area is more easily released. This is called the Bohr Effect, and was discovered by Danish physiologist Dr Bohr and friends in 1904. While the Bohr Effect seems odd at first glance, it has great utility in that, at different times, different organs and muscles will be working harder than others, and as they do so the oxygen they have converts to energy and CO_2, so more CO_2 is released and then more oxygen is taken up at exactly those places in the body that need it. It is a mechanism of the body to efficiently deliver oxygen where it is needed most.

This is great for efficient delivery of oxygen where it is needed — but there is a downside. Breathing a lot more than we need to, such as hyperventilating when at rest, means that more CO_2 is breathed out, leading to a general drop in CO_2. If we breathe too much when not actually doing physical activity that requires it, CO_2 levels drop. Overbreathing doesn't really affect the oxygen levels as the haemoglobin usually fills to close to maximum quite quickly; but it does affect carbon dioxide as there is much more CO_2 dissolved in the blood and it can keep being exchanged, hence the level can be lowered.

Lower carbon dioxide equates to more alkaline blood. This matters because it especially affects the brain, where overbreathing means less carbon dioxide, which in turn means blood vessels constrict and so less blood flows. It seems this constriction is especially pronounced in the brain. (This is thought to also be due to interactions with the cerebrospinal fluid.) The low carbon dioxide also reduces the release of oxygen, due to the Bohr Effect. This point is so counterintuitive that it is worth explaining in more detail because, in short, it means that if you breathe too much your brain gets less oxygen. Up to a certain point, the more oxygen you breathe in, the more oxygen gets to your brain and body, and you may need to breathe harder when doing physical work. Overbreathing at rest or in general life is quite common, however, and the harder you breathe, the more carbon dioxide is exhaled; so, too little CO_2 means the blood vessels contract and carry less blood. Also, when the blood reaches its destination less oxygen is exchanged. So two mechanisms mean overbreathing leads to less oxygen being available to the brain.

These mechanisms explain why the old-fashioned remedy of breathing into a paper bag works when someone is hyperventilating — because this brings up the CO_2 level, and once this is raised the blood vessels of the brain expand again and the oxygen–carbon dioxide exchange is re-established. However, breathing into a paper bag is no longer recommended because if you do too much of it you can go the other extreme of not enough oxygen, which is much worse.

The best breathing for optimal oxygenation is about balance. Underbreathing is a problem, but so is overbreathing.

Given that most people think that carbon dioxide is just a waste product, it can be surprising to see the range of important roles it plays. As well as playing a crucial role in maintaining the correct pH level of the blood, CO_2 also does the following:

- **It acts to relax the smooth muscles in the walls of our blood vessels, and as such assists in blood flow and the transport of oxygen.**

- It relaxes the muscles in the gastrointestinal tract, and as such helps digestion in the gut, minimizing potential problems such as irritable bowel syndrome.
- Relaxing the smooth muscles also occurs in the airways, so CO_2 acts as a natural bronchodilator, assisting effective breathing.
- It relaxes the smooth muscles of the bladder and uterus, helping them function optimally.
- It plays important roles in the synthesis and function of antibodies, hormones and enzyme.
- It has a calming effect on the nervous system.[1]

Basically, we need carbon dioxide. It is a crucial chemical for proper functioning of many of the body's systems and not enough of it creates problems.

Importantly, though, too much of it is also a problem, quite independently of how much oxygen we have. If people underbreathe (due to medical lung conditions, for example, or with some forms of depression) not enough carbon dioxide is exchanged and the blood and cellular fluids become more acidic. This can have a chain of reactions on cell function, including being likely to reduce responsivity of brain function. This is not so much of a surprise, as most people would expect too much CO_2 to be a problem, but some of the many ways it is problematic are still being mapped out.[2]

So carbon dioxide is crucial, we just need it in the right balance.

... and nitric oxide is part of the gang

Nitric oxide is another important molecule linked with the breath. While not so critical as oxygen, in everyday life nitric oxide has a range of important functions in many body systems, and especially has a role in dilating blood vessels.

In the early 1990s it was discovered that enzymes in the nose, and especially in the paranasal sinuses, produce nitric oxide, and in 1998 the Nobel Prize for Physiology or Medicine was awarded to Robert Furchgott, Louis Ignarro and Ferid Murad for discovering the way that nitric oxide acts as a unique signalling molecule in the cardiovascular system. Since then its role in many other systems has also been studied.[3]

Low nitric oxide levels in the body are associated with a range of disorders including heart disease, diabetes, erectile dysfunction and dementia. Raising nitric oxide levels in the bloodstream is protective against these disorders and many medical sources will recommend eating foods rich in nitrogen or taking supplements to help with this. It is less widely known that breathing through the nose also has a powerful effect in increasing nitric oxide levels.

Nitric oxide:

- **increases vasodilation and hence acts to reduce high blood pressure**
- **has an anti-inflammatory action**
- **has an important function in strengthening immunity and fighting infection**
- **enables or enhances erectile function**
- **enhances memory and learning**
- **acts as a signalling molecule and as a hormone for maintaining many normal body functions.**[4]

So, long-term, keeping up levels of nitric oxide is very important for general health, and breathing through the nose raises these levels. Short-term, the immediate vasodilation effect is a reason why breathing through the nose leads to feeling more alert and clear-headed. Slow breathing through the nose seems to enhance the effect.

Another reason to breathe through the nose — it's the **Nitric Oxide System Enhancer**.

Breathing and embodied alarm systems: fight or flight vs calm states

Breathing can play a big role in many body functions.

The nervous system has two main systems outside of the brain and spinal cord: the somatic nervous system, which involves control over all our voluntary muscles, such as in walking, talking or exercising; and the autonomic nervous system, which controls all the organs and is mostly not under conscious control. Breathing can obviously play a role in exercise, and most people who go to a gym will learn to coordinate movement with breath to get better results. What is less obvious is that the breath can also give some measure of control over other body functions.

Two of our most basic and pervasive modes are the fight or flight response and the calm mode (sometimes also called 'rest and digest' or 'relax and repair'). These are 'wired in' to us through evolution and happen at the autonomic nervous system level, which in turn has two main systems: one which speeds things up (the sympathetic nervous system) and the other which calms things down (the parasympathetic nervous system). Mammals, including humans, are geared to mostly be in a more relaxed mode — to forage, do simple work, play, eat, rest and digest (which is linked to the parasympathetic nervous system). If you imagine a group of chimps eating, grooming or resting, it is that mode.

The other mode is being activated, switched on to react and fully alert. This can be helpful for many activities, from playing sport to engaging in anything exciting. When everyday life is enjoyable there is usually some balance of activation and relaxation. The activation mode, though, is fully switched on in response to threat. In this mode (the sympathetic nervous system) we need to react to threats to survival. If you suddenly sense you are in great danger, a number of changes happen. Imagine strolling through the jungle and coming face to face with a tiger. Adrenaline and noradrenaline are released. This helps you move more quickly and strongly. Cortisol is released, which helps the body produce more immediate energy so you can run away. The brain also goes into something of a short circuit, so those sections that help you sense danger and move quickly are maximized, while large parts of the brain linked with, say, language and creativity are made more 'offline' because the emphasis is on survival and they aren't needed right now. Blood flow also changes, away from the gut to the arms and legs (there's no point digesting your lunch if you're about to become someone else's). When all of this happens the body is geared for major physical action, and when we then take major physical action, like running away very fast, this acts to burn off and flush through the stress chemicals, which shift us out of that state. (Think of the gazelles on a nature documentary, who bound away when they see a leopard but 20 minutes later are happily grazing again.)

This 'survival mode' links with fight or flight and has been very successful in an evolutionary sense. The response means that if the predator is bigger than us we can run away faster and if we are cornered we can fight harder.

This works well in the jungle. However, when we get stressed about work or modern life our bodies go through the same types of physiological response (even if to a lesser degree). The fight or flight reaction is designed for short bursts, and when we stay stressed it has harmful effects on our health. Exercise is a great way to burn off and flush through the adrenaline and cortisol produced by this stress response. The other simple and immediate way to shift out of this mode is slow, deep diaphragmatic breathing.

Being long-term in the sympathetic nervous system mode — the fight or flight response brought about by stress — leads to a huge range of health problems, so learning to shift into a calming response has huge benefits for health and healing.

Zoe

Zoe was distressed as she talked to me. She was an overseas student, and her family had worked hard to help give her the opportunity to study overseas. Two months earlier she had found out her father had cancer. Initially, everyone had kept the information from her, not wanting her studies to be affected. Eventually she found out and was deeply worried and feeling profoundly alone in a foreign county. She knew his cancer was likely to be terminal but no one would say anything other than that he was responding well to treatment.

Zoe had been completely unable to focus on her studies but felt compelled to pretend she was progressing well whenever she had contact with home. As she fell further behind, she felt more lonely and desperate. Her supervisor convinced her to get help, and in the session with me she was caught in high pitched sobs, barely able to talk and feeling overwhelmed. Usually, in a therapy session, once someone has been able to describe what has happened and feel understood they calm a little, but Zoe was so caught in this agitated, anxious distress that she did not calm, so we focused on breathing. I explained that taking some slow, deep breaths would help her be more in charge of the emotion. I asked her to place one hand on her belly. Then when breathing out I asked her to squeeze her abdominal muscles, gently pushing her hand in to aid the feeling of it, so as to extend the out-breath. Given that she had been crying so much, she could not breathe through her nose, so I asked her to purse her lips as if breathing through a straw. She was able to do this and began to breathe more slowly and deeply. This produced a clear change as she moved out of the distressed (sympathetic nervous system) state and into a more relaxed state. I asked how she felt doing this and she said 'calm'. For most of the session she had looked at the floor but now she lifted her gaze and looked at me. This changed happened within a couple of minutes and was profound.

As we talked further, Zoe would sometimes slip back into agitation and distress, but each time we could use this purposeful breathing to come back to a calmer state once again. We could begin to talk more clearly about how to best respond to the difficulties she faced. Of course, the breathing did not solve the difficulties, but it enabled her to clearly think through her best options for responding to the situation. It helped her to move out of the distressed, fight or flight state into a calmer mode.

Signs you're calm or in fight or flight mode

There can be visible signs and sensations of either the fight or flight mode, or calmer mode while dealing with difficult emotions. In therapy, when people are talking through traumas or other distressing events, it is much more therapeutic to be out of the sympathetic mode, which can feel retraumatizing.

The following lists draw on the work of trauma therapist Sue Hetzel.[5] A list like this is helpful when helping others, but can also be a reference for cues to your own states.

Signs of sympathetic nervous system activation (being the fight or flight mode) include:

- dry mouth/difficulty swallowing
- pale skin
- increased heart rate (pulse)
- cooler skin/hands, cold sweat
- large pupils
- crying on inhalation, high pitched voice
- rapid, shallow breathing, panting, inhaling quickly
- increased muscle tone
- mind racing, worrying.

Signs of parasympathetic nervous system activation include:

- sighs/deep exhale
- flushed skin colour
- slower heart rate (pulse)
- dry skin, usually warm to touch
- small pupils
- soft crying
- slower, deeper respiration
- reduced/relaxed muscle tone
- clearer thinking.

Freeze

As well as fight/flight or calm modes, an important third mode is the freeze response. This, too, is an important survival mechanism that has worked in evolution. In this response, if the predator is bigger and faster than us, the body can shut down into a freeze state. If you have seen a mouse caught by a cat, the mouse can appear dead. It is not 'playing possum' in the sense of making a decision to pretend to be dead; the freeze response has taken over, making the mouse limp and apparently lifeless. 'Freezing' has been an important last defence in evolution as sometimes the predator loses interest, while at other times it helps the potential victim remain unnoticed. It also helps to survive the trauma, and in humans is linked with dissociation. People who have been assaulted sometimes wonder why they froze and didn't fight back — the freezing response is a deeply embodied defensive reaction.

How this response happens has been illuminated by Stephen Porges, creator of 'polyvagal theory'. He described the roles played by the vagus nerve, which plays a central role in the parasympathetic nervous system.[6] The word 'vagus' comes from the Latin and means 'wandering', and this nerve is our longest cranial nerve connecting the brain and many different organ systems.

The vagus nerve appears to have developed over the course of evolution, and has an older section which connects especially with the gut, and a newer section which connects with the muscles of the face, voice and middle ear. The gut part remains more primitive in structure (not having the myelination or sheathing of the nerves that the more recent system has). The more primitive vagus is linked with digestion and also with switching on a primitive defensive response of 'freezing'. The newer section connects to the muscles of the face and voice. As mammals evolved they increasingly lived in groups and their survival depended on the group's harmony and ability to coordinate interactions. Facial expressions and voice tone became ways to regulate bonding or responses to threat. In humans and other mammals, the higher connection to face and voice means we can often soothe ourselves and others through facial expression and tone of voice. A smile and

41

warmth in vocal tone helps the person with whom we're interacting to feel calm, relaxed and connected. Neuroscientists call this downregulating the threat response.

While these social responses can calm down threat reactions, if the situation is too threatening then the fight or flight reactions take over. These reactions activate you to take defensive action, but if you are in a situation of life threat in which you can neither get away nor win the fight, the more primitive vagal system can kick in and the freeze response can take over. So there are three basic states described here: first, the social engagement system linked with calm states of safety; second, the (sympathetic) fight or flight; and third, an immobilizing 'freeze' response.

There can be a chain of response: if our talking and facial expressions do not stop a threat, the sympathetic (fight or flight) response kicks in, speeding up breathing and heart rate so we can react more quickly or strongly; and if this is overwhelmed, the freeze response can take over. Thankfully this does not happen often, but it does happen at times when people are exposed to traumatic events or unable to escape threats to their survival.

The other aspect to add here is that polyvagal theory also explains more about positive states of mobilization. In friendly interactions, such as sports, the social engagement system is engaged at the same time as sympathetic activation, so there can be a safe and positive activation.

Importantly, the vagus nerve is also linked with the breath. The calming response can also be switched on with deep diaphragmatic breathing and slow exhalations.

Neuroception: reacting faster than you can think

For issues such as managing anxiety, it helps to know that mind–body reactions often happen faster than we can think.

'Neuroception' is perception that happens outside of conscious awareness, particularly an immediate reaction to threat. Mood states, especially anxiety states, are often kicked off quickly outside of conscious awareness, and then we try to catch up and figure out what happened.

Understanding a bit about the brain's structure helps make sense of this. The brain has many sections — in some ways it is as if we have many different brains, rather than just one. These smaller brains don't always work together well. They each have different functions and different sections take charge at different times. Our evolutionary processes have geared us to prioritize survival (the processes that didn't prioritize survival probably aren't around anymore).

There are three main parts to the brain, which have developed through evolution; this model of the brain is called the 'triune' brain. At the top of the spinal cord and at the base of the brain is the brain stem, which is sometimes called the reptilian brain. The brain stem, the first part of the brain to develop, controls basic bodily functions such as heartbeat. On top of, and around, the brain stem is the 'mammalian brain' or limbic system, which has many parts related to emotion, motivation and embodied learning. This links to many of the complex social bonding and relationships that are found in groups of mammals. Around that is the 'neo-mammalian brain', which has the bigger cortex and frontal areas that are most pronounced in humans and allow higher learning, mathematics and remembering the shopping list.

One of the key parts of the brain is the amygdala, at the front of the limbic system. The amygdala is the brain's 'alarm system' and is wired to respond very quickly to signs of threat. After a trauma the amygdala can often stay over-sensitized to anything that looks like a threat. It is designed to keep us safe but can be a problem when it goes off too often. This works well in evolution. If you are out walking and see a brown stick, the amygdala might have you jump backwards, heart racing and ready to run. If it is just a brown stick the response is a bit inconvenient but if it is a deadly snake, the amygdala just saved you.

The problem for many people is that the amygdala works too well after a trauma. Soldiers coming back from combat might go into full fight or flight mode when a car backfires. Someone who was beaten up by an attacker wearing a red coat might react to any piece of red clothing. If you had a terrible experience presenting to a group, any group situation might trigger things off.

One of the important things to know is that the alarm system happens faster than we can think. The amygdala reacts in about 1/20 of a second. By contrast, the hippocampus (which is involved in long-term learning and does the job of sorting out whether it really is a snake or a stick) takes about half a second. Actually thinking it all through consciously takes longer again.

Often, the amygdala 'hijacks' the brain and we respond to threat before we are aware of why. Sometimes people with anxiety or post-traumatic difficulties feel as if they respond in irrational ways to some things, but the 'amygdala hijack' is often the reason. Recognizing this means it is easier to respond to it and get the rest of the brain back online.

Most people have a 'default mode' when faced with a threatening situation, including social threats such as rejection. Some people get anxious, some might withdraw, others may become depressed or have 'somaticized' (body) responses such as feeling weighed down and physically worn out. All of these reactions and modes may be kicked off faster than we realize, and are associational rather than rational. We might react to someone else who looks a bit like the person who attacked us, or to a voice tone. Recognizing this means we can learn to change it over time.

Sympathetic nervous system states are often triggered without us being consciously aware of it, and part of our response is also an immediate change in breathing pattern. If we notice we have been thrown into one of these anxiety states, we can take control of our breathing to shift the pattern, and with it influence the mood and mode — this might not fully change the mode but can at least ease the anxiety, or boost a sense of feeling centred, so we can decide how best to respond. It puts us back in charge — calmer, stronger, centred and more able to decide how best to respond.

Interoception: developing a core intelligence

I always like discoveries in psychology that help me to feel smarter, and one of the areas that has had recent focus is the range of people's intelligence. Traditional notions of intelligence have focused on a narrow range of abilities, such as the use of language, solving academic puzzles, speed of processing information and how much we can hold in our head while sorting out problems.

Recent years have seen an increased focus on multiple intelligence, which includes musical and artistic abilities, and athletic capacities.[7] Emotional intelligence has become highly valued, recognizing both our own emotions and our responsiveness to the feelings of and interactions with others. This is now often seen as more important than traditional intelligence in areas such as management.

One other area that all of us have always had to some extent, but which has not always been clearly identified, is *interoception*. This is the intelligence of being aware of what is happening in our bodies. It is distinct from proprioception, which is awareness of how we are moving our limbs or holding ourselves in space. It is an intelligence of inner awareness.

This inner awareness might be of feelings in our gut, of muscles contracting, of the need to move after sitting for a time, of our heart rate or our breathing. As neurophysiologist Clare J. Fowler has stated, 'The system of interoception as a whole constitutes *the material me* and relates to how we perceive feelings from our bodies that determine our mood, sense of well-being and emotions'.[8] Being able to recognize more subtle levels of what is happening in our bodies enables us to enlist more fully the intelligence of the body, and enables a sense of being in the body in a way that is grounded and integrated. In contrast, people who have gone through severely traumatic experiences can dissociate and disconnect from bodily experience. The body can become unknown and unpredictable and feel as if it is hostile. If your body is acting in unpredictable ways, life is likely to feel very unsafe. Gently regaining awareness of the body, through practices such as trauma-sensitive yoga, allows new avenues of comfort and safety.

More generally, awareness of the breath is a form of interoception. By simply doing any of the exercises in this book, you can develop more subtle levels of awareness of the breathing and body. The breath can be a pathway to feeling at home in the body. For some, feeling at home in their bodies may feel so normal and natural that it seems a strange concept to name, but for many people this simple comfort is blocked. Most of us grow up in cultures that foster mind over body and pushing the body to achieve goals rather than really listening to it. Bodies are often treated as machines, and we can become trained to disconnect. Ignoring the body can also lead to ignoring the warning signs of medical conditions.

Slow deep breathing can foster a sense of calm and be a simple way to also be focused within, in body awareness. This can both build interoception and allow one of the simplest of pleasures, that of relaxing and being 'comfortable in your own skin'.

A simple practice can be to take a few slow deep breaths and then to close your eyes and allow the awareness to spread through your body, just noticing whatever sensations are there. (See the exercise 'Full breath with passive exhalation on p. 68.)

Heart rate variability

Breathing is linked to the function of the heart. While it is easy to think of the heart as having a steady beat, a healthy heart actually changes the rate of beating in response to a whole range of stimuli, and subtle changes to the interval between heart beats occurs. If this change in heart rate is not present and the heartbeat remains too fixed, it is a sign of potential ill health, stress related disorders and a range of psychiatric disorders. Of course, a wildly erratic heartbeat would be even worse, but regular variation is very healthy.

The heartbeat will speed up a bit with an inhalation and slow down a bit with an exhalation. You can test this simply for yourself by finding your pulse (in your wrist or neck) then feeling the count of the heartbeat as you take some slow deep breaths. The change is subtle but the heart rate should speed up a bit as you inhale and slow down a bit as you exhale. This change is known as *respiratory sinus arrhythmia*. On the inhalation the sympathetic activating nervous system is more pronounced and on the exhalation the calming (parasympathetic) system is more active. The main mechanism for this is that a healthy vagus nerve will act as a 'vagal brake' on the heart rate during the exhalation. If the vagal nerve mechanism is not working well (what is referred to as poor vagal tone) the heart rate stays high.

If you are chronically stressed or have suffered severe trauma, the system can be thrown out and heart rate varies little. More technically, Stephen Porges describes that 'When we inhale, the influence of the vagus is weakened and the heart rate increases. When we breathe out, the influence of the vagus becomes stronger and the heart rate sinks. This simple mechanical change during breathing strengthens the calming and generally positive impact of the myelinated vagus on the body'.[9] This cycle of slight speeding up and slowing down of the heart rate is central to good health — in particular by reducing stress states.

Slow breathing is very important: the breath needs to be slow enough to allow the vagal brake to work. If you are breathing at fifteen or 20 breaths per minute there is very little chance for the vagal brake to work and the heart rate stays high and relatively unchanged, meaning you stay in a stressed fight or flight state.

Slower breathing allows the change of the rate of the heart to occur in a regular fashion, which reflects harmony in the body. A heart that has these regular changes is much more able to respond to challenges — to speed up in times of stress and slow down in recovery.

Psychotherapist Wilfried Ehrmann has summarized a range of studies suggesting that when the heart is in this dynamic balance:

- blood pressure is lower
- less energy is consumed
- the ageing process slows
- there are improvements in immunity
- susceptibility for fears and depression is reduced
- emotional coping with the challenges of life is improved.[10]

To achieve the best outcome of a regular changing of the heart rate, a range of recent research has suggested that breathing should be slowed down to about five or six breaths per minute.[11]

Life energy: *chi, ki, prana*

Life energy, or life force, has long been recognized as something crucial to good health, healing and vitality. In Japanese martial arts it is referred to as *ki*, in Chinese systems such as tai chi and *chi kung* it is called *chi* and in yoga the term *prana* means both life energy and the energy of the breath. Anyone practising these traditions for a while will have no doubt about the reality of this life force, but while powerful it is also subtle and there is no accepted Western equivalent for these terms. Some Western philosophers accept it, and in Russia there are longstanding claims that it can be photographed with *kirlian* photography, but it is not yet recognized in Western science.[12]

Breathing well can be used to boost energy within a few breaths, and breathing patterns can enhance vitality. There are important explanations for this in Western science, including increased oxygen levels, increased blood flow, better muscle function, subtle shifts of biochemistry and hormone balances. All of these correlate with *prana*, but to anyone who practises Eastern techniques it is clear that there is an immediate effect of breathing on life force that has not yet been fully explained in the West. While this might sound foreign to you, I ask that you hold an open mind to notice your own experience as you try some of the exercises in the book. Breathing can be used purposefully to boost energy levels and restore balance.

4

PROBLEM BREATHING

Many problematic patterns of breathing are a response to stress, difficult emotions or trauma — the body reacts and gets stuck in particular patterns. Other problematic patterns may just be bad habits. While typical patterns are described below, it is important to remember that some breathing problems may also be a response to underlying medical conditions and what is outlined below is not intended to substitute for individual assessment by your medical practitioner.

As you read these patterns, if you feel that your own breathing is abnormal, please get a medical check, and when trying the exercises in this book never force anything — all the exercises should be practised gently.

Overbreathing

One common form of problem breathing is overbreathing.

Normal breathing is usually considered to be about eight to twelve breaths per minute. Normal volume of the breath is about 500 to 600 ml per breath, so in one minute about 5 or 6 litres of air are inhaled and exhaled. Not all of this breath is used, as some stays in the airways and doesn't reach the alveoli for gas exchange. A normal breath (around 500 ml) is not a huge amount so there is not much noticeable movement of the chest or belly.

Importantly, there is quite a lot of reserve volume in the lungs, so we can take in more air if we need to, such as during exercise.

Many people breathe too much volume or too rapidly, and this constitutes overbreathing. Breathing through the mouth means much more air is likely to go in and out. Deep, repeated sighs can also be part of this, as a deep sigh can be 2 or even 3 litres of air. Rates of breathing also are part of overbreathing. While ten to fourteen breaths per minute at rest is considered normal, more than fifteen will usually be overbreathing.

Over the years there have been many medical reports of chronic overbreathing, which has been called 'hyperventilation syndrome'. Reports of this go back to at least the American Civil War but have been especially collated and described in a series of books by Robert Fried.[1] Hyperventilation can potentially produce a wide range of symptoms and related conditions including: fatigue, weakness, exhaustion, palpitations, rapid pulse, chest pain, cold, numbness or tingling in the fingers and toes, dizziness, lightheadedness, disturbance of consciousness or vision, shortness of breath, dry mouth, yawning, a lump in the throat, pain below the ribs (epigastric pain), burping, muscle pains, cramps and spasms, tremors, stiffness, anxiety, insomnia and nightmares.[2] Fried highlights that periodically over the decades these types of symptoms have been identified as being caused by overbreathing. Indeed, it is curious that something that has been 'rediscovered' over and over again over many decades is so under-recognized, and Fried has been a passionate campaigner to have hyperventilation more recognized in general medical practice. Of note, most of the symptoms of anxiety disorders may be linked to overbreathing. Reports suggest that up to 10 per cent of the population may suffer from this.[3] Panic attacks and sleep apnoea may also be caused by overbreathing. If sleep apnoea is caused by it, it is also worth being aware that since there is such an extremely high correlation between sleep apnoea and depression, it could be a significant contributor to many cases of depression.[4]

Reverse breathing

When breathing diaphragmatically, the diaphragm contracts, pulling downwards so the belly moves out a little on the inhalation and moves back in on the exhalation. Breathing in, the belly goes out; breathing out, the belly goes in.

In reverse breathing, the opposite happens. The breath is taken mostly into the chest and as this happens the belly moves in. On the out-breath the chest moves and the belly falls outward. In this style of breathing the breath is mostly controlled by the rib muscles and upper chest muscles, and the diaphragm is barely engaged at all. For anyone used to breathing correctly it is quite uncomfortable, but it is surprisingly common.

Because reverse breathing overuses the muscles of the chest, upper chest and often shoulders to compensate for barely using the diaphragm, it can lead to a lot of tension, not just in the chest and shoulders but throughout the body. It also leads to tiredness, as some muscles become exhausted from overuse and because the breath is not efficient. It can contribute to gastrointestinal problems because the organs of the belly are not getting the natural movement and massage that occurs with diaphragmatic breathing. The unnatural nature of reverse breathing can also lead to difficulty in coordination, as it is at odds with natural movement.

'Natural' movement of the breath can be observed in young children. If you watch a two- or three-year-old lying down resting, perhaps drifting off to sleep; what moves most is their belly, in tune with the diaphragm. Their belly goes out as they breathe in, and in as they breathe out. For many of us, this is lost at some point when growing up.

In my experience, most people, when asked to take a deep breath, will consciously breathe into their chest, and many will breathe into the upper chest, lifting up their shoulders and not engaging the diaphragm. It is as if we adults think that the lungs are up there, and that the upper chest is what has to work. Since the diaphragm is not visible (and the ribcage is) many of us just focus on the ribcage when consciously breathing. This fits with the pattern of reverse breathing.

Dan

Dan saw me for help with chronic tension, tiredness and low-level depression. He had seen counsellors before and when we talked, he told me of events that might have led to him feeling depressed. He was very active and played regular sport. We discussed breathing and when I asked him to take a deep breath, he clearly had a big lung capacity and his chest swelled impressively, but his diaphragm was not engaged. He had a clear pattern of reverse breathing.

When we began to practise diaphragmatic breathing it was initially hard for him to 'get it', but he had excellent body awareness so managed it before long, and agreed to practise. It had a calming effect on him and over time helped with general mood and energy levels. Many reverse breathers also find it helps with sports and coordination, when they shift to breathing more diaphragmatically.

High breathing

High breathing is breathing to the upper chest. It can be both a cause and effect of anxiety.

Most people, if they get a sudden shock such as seeing a snake on the path, will take a short sharp intake of breath into the top of the lungs. If the threat remains they will tend to breathe out very little and breathe in again to the upper chest. This links with the fight or flight response and is not a problem if it happens for a few moments when under threat.

For many people, though, this way of breathing becomes habitual. I see it very often in people who come for help with anxiety. The diaphragm barely moves and is effectively 'frozen'. When asked to take a deep breath the person will lift up even more into the upper chest and can't take much in because their exhalation has been so restricted — as if the lower two-thirds of the lungs don't get used. While it could be called 'chest breathing', it really involves the upper chest and muscles linked to the shoulders. People who habitually breathe this way tend to carry a lot of tension in their bodies. This might lead to tension headaches or at least a lot of tightness in the neck and shoulders. It also affects the abdominal organs because the diaphragm is frozen, so no natural movement happens with the breath.

High breathing can play a big part in the development of hypertension, which in turn can link to heart disease, circulatory issues and risk for strokes.

Frozen breathing

Other patterns can greatly restrict the breath.

After being under threat, wild animals are likely to run away or fight if cornered, and it seems their bodies reset after the stress or trauma. Even if they become immobilized, if they survive they run off and reset. On the other hand, recent research suggests that humans under threat often cannot run off in the same way and that our systems often do not reset properly, but maintain a degree of the response that happened under threat.[5] Some of these threats may be physical but many may be social, and there may be a suppression of response, including a freezing-up of the breath, as the best way of getting through at the time. Interestingly, while wild animals seem to reset themselves after threat, caged animals may not, and a study in which rats were placed under repeated social stress (being put in other cages with dominant rats) showed many of them had a repressed breathing rate for weeks afterwards.[6]

While the cause may not always be known, some people can have a very frozen breathing pattern with hardly any noticeable breathing movement. There is also a high level of tension, as opposed to a relaxed but small, gentle breath which also may not produce much visible motion. The difference is the tension, and any small movement will usually be high in the chest.

Collapsed breathing

Other people can have such a slumped posture that it is almost impossible for them to breathe properly. The lungs are compressed and the belly slumps forward. This is sometimes due to depression, but must in itself contribute to depression, as the breathing restriction chronically flattens energy.

If you let yourself slump forward as you are reading this, you'll immediately feel that it becomes much harder to breathe fully. Breathing in becomes an effort and breathing out is just letting go. It promotes a tendency to pause before breathing in again. It is not hard to imagine that this posture and this restricted style of breathing can link with depression ... and if you have tried this while you are reading, notice the difference if you sit upright and open the upper chest as you next breathe in.

Reactive or habitual breathing

As well as those styles listed above, there is a range of breathing styles that vary with individuals, including jerky breath or breathing with frequent sighs or yawning.

Changes of breathing pattern under conditions of stress or of exertion, such as exercise, are mostly a good thing, as this is part of being responsive to the demands of the moment. The main point is awareness. It is often hard to stop and focus on your breathing in a stressful situation, as most of the time you will focus on the stress — there is no point stopping to notice your breathing if a truck is about to run you over. On the other hand, if you know you regularly become anxious, say, in social situations, then controlling the breath can be a very helpful way to calm down (as will be outlined in the chapters to follow).

The best breathing is flexible, responding to the particular demands of the moment, while also having the best everyday baseline pattern. Some researchers suggest that as much as two-thirds of the population either overbreathe or underbreathe.[7] If you can be more aware of your own breathing patterns, you can then be more in charge of your breathing, including by using some of the breathing styles outlined in Chapter 6.

PART 2

Getting started

5

KEY PRINCIPLES OF PURPOSEFUL BREATHING

When using the breath as a way to change mood and energy level, there are a few principles to bear in mind that are helpful, and which inform the styles of breathing for particular purposes in the section that follows.

Do something different

There are whole approaches to therapy based on the principle of 'When there is a problem, *do something different*'. The same applies to breathing. If you want to change how you are feeling, take a moment to notice your breathing and change it. If your breathing is fast and shallow, make it slower and deeper. If it is jumpy, make it even, and so on.

- **Breathing deep and diaphragmatically** rather than high in the chest has a calming effect.
- **The slower the breath the more calming it is,** as long as it stays reasonably comfortable, of course, not so slow as to be

forced or make you short of breath.

- **Extending the exhalation is calming.** Longer exhalations activate the relaxation response of the body.
- **Having the in- and out-breaths about the same length also helps bring a sense of being calm and centred.** Although it is a subtle effect, having the in-breath longer than the out-breath tends to raise people's energy, and having the out-breath longer than the in-breath tends to lower energy. While you can choose to have longer exhalations to relax or longer inhalation to energize, keeping it even is usually simple and helpful.
- **Breathing in and out for about five or six seconds each brings balance.** The length of the breath is important. In general, the slower you breathe the calmer the effect of the breathing, as long as you stay within comfortable limits — if you force it to be too slow it will be uncomfortable, and then you'll tense up. When you stop to focus on the breath, an ideal is to breathe for about five or six breaths per minute. This seems to strike a special resonance, a 'sweet spot' that brings a range of physical factors into balance.

Holding your breath

Often when people have strong, difficult emotions they unconsciously hold the breath, so it is better to **be aware not to hold the breath, unless for a specific purpose.** Instead, move from the in-breath to the out-breath, and the out-breath to the in-breath with only a relaxed, natural gap in between. Holding the breath in or out tends to hold the emotional state of the moment. Breath holding, if you do it, should be careful and deliberate. If you are feeling down, for example, holding the breath may lift you up, and if overbreathing, then pausing after the exhalation will help restore the CO_2 and O_2 balance.

Focus on the breath

Focusing on the breath in itself tends to help with calming and centring because it helps to redirect the mind. When people are anxious they typically have a lot of anxious thoughts, which then feed the anxiety. Focusing on the breath helps to interrupt this by moving you from a self-talk mode to a sensing mode.

Inhale to raise energy, exhale to lower energy

While in a literal sense the inhalation and exhalation must balance overall in volume, the length and focus of the breath make a difference. When the inhalation is longer than the exhalation it tends to raise energy in the body. When the exhalation is longer it tends to lower energy. This happens spontaneously in people feeling anxious or depressed and they can consciously change it. Most of the time you will want balance, so will probably want your inhalation and exhalation to be about the same length. However, if you are feeling flat you can lengthen the inhalation, breathing in for, say, a count of eight and out for a count of four. Make sure to keep within comfortable limits, not forcing the inhalation. If you are feeling overstimulated, anxious or on edge, you might lengthen the exhalation, breathing out for, say, a count of eight and in for a count of four.

Breathing to the front is more emotional; breathing to the back is more calming

The breath can be directed to the front of the body, the back or more to the centre.

If you breathe to the front of the body, it tends to be more emotional. You might want this if you have felt emotionally 'blocked'. Breathing to the back tends to be more calming and more meditative. You can also consciously breathe so as to fill up the centre of the body. This is balanced and good for general activity.

Breath can link with posture

Bending forward is calming, while opening the chest (bending back) is energizing.

Linked with the notion of breathing to the front or the back of the body is the practice of opening the front or the back more with movement. When you open the front of the body, such as by a yoga style backbend, it is energizing. When you do a forward bend, opening the back of the body and closing in the front, it tends to be calming. In daily life, you tend to see posture reflect this. Depressed people are often slumped in their posture, with the front of the body closed and held in. Changing posture and opening the chest helps to lift mood and energize, such as with the old-fashioned advice to stand tall with shoulders back.

Holding the breath tends to hold or block energy

People who are depressed often sigh the breath out and unconsciously hold the breath out. People who are very stressed and having difficulty with a particular emotion often hold the breath, inadvertently blocking the emotion.

We've probably all heard the phrase when facing a difficult challenge to 'take a deep breath' and then just do it. In practice, when people do this they often take the deep breath, then hold it a little. This lifts the energy and helps them step forward.

For people who are going through grief or depression, taking a deep breath and holding it lifts them a little. It is surprisingly difficult to stay quite so 'down' when you are holding a large full breath.

On the other hand, in therapy, people who are dealing with other powerful emotions often literally stop breathing for significant periods. Gently encouraging them to keep breathing allows them to work through the emotion more effectively.

Breathing can be soft and gentle or strong and muscular

Each of these breathing styles produces different effects, to be more calming or more energizing.

Learning to breathe in a strong, muscular fashion is now a part of many athletes' training regimes. Some approaches use an apparatus to provide resistance against the breath so the athlete has to work harder to get the breath in. In doing this the diaphragm is always central but the full range of chest and abdominal muscles can be engaged to add strength and endurance. The aim of course, is that in those last minutes of the race or the game the athlete can breathe more strongly so as to compete better.

The best breathing is balanced breathing

While best breathing will be responsive and vary according to the demands of the moment, in general the best breathing is balanced. It is not about breathing as hard or as fully as you can — it is easy to overbreathe. A sweet spot happens where the breath is slow and even, which leads to a sense of physical, mental and emotional balance.

6

BREATHING STYLES AND BASIC TECHNIQUES

The breathing styles detailed in this chapter are mostly simple and available to everyone. You need to breathe anyway, so you might as well do it consciously to reap the greater benefits.

Cautions and contraindications

One if the central points of this book is that slow, deep breathing done with awareness is great for feeling calmer and stronger. It promotes a sense of being centred and is also great for general health.

There are a few important exceptions. First, breathing patterns can be thrown out by an underlying medical condition, so if any of the exercises in this book feel uncomfortable, don't force anything and make sure to get a medical check-up. I have taught these techniques to hundreds of people in my work as a psychologist, but many of these have been referred by doctors who have already ruled out medical causes (for say, panic attacks), and if there is any doubt I always err on the side of caution and recommend a check-up first.

Difficulties can also arise for people who have suffered trauma. While learning conscious breathing is a huge help for overcoming post-traumatic symptoms, if you have had an experience of suffocating, then controlling the breath may initially raise some anxiety, so go gently with it. In his work on trauma-sensitive yoga, David Emerson gives an example of working with a former sniper who had been trained to pull the trigger on a long, slow exhalation; for him, a slow exhalation brought up post-traumatic reactions.[1]

Occasionally, a person can have what is called a paradoxical reaction to relaxing. If you have suffered abuse at times of being relaxed, that association can be triggered. This is rare, but can happen.

Do everything in the book gently — I do not suggest doing anything that is uncomfortable — with awareness and to your own comfort limits.

BELLY BREATHING

'Belly breathing' is often the quickest and easiest way for many people to use their diaphragm. It produces a sense of being calm and centred.

Sit with a straight back and with your feet on the floor, and place one hand on your chest and one hand over the navel. As you breathe, notice which hand moves more: with your inhalation or exhalation? Many people typically chest breathe, so that during an inhalation the hand on the chest moves outward more than the other hand.

For belly breathing the simple guideline is: **breathing in, the belly goes out; breathing out, the belly goes in.**

To get the feeling of this, it helps to actively use the muscles of your abdomen on the exhalation, squeezing in the belly to squeeze the air out. It can also help to gently push in on the belly with the hand when breathing out — this focuses attention there and helps you get used to the movement. On the in-breath, don't push the belly out at all; just allow it to relax as it moves with the breath.

Belly breathing is relatively easily learnt, even when people are highly anxious, and has a calming effect. Once you are more practised at belly breathing the focus will move to the diaphragm. The belly should gently and passively move out on the inhalation as the diaphragm contracts and pulls down. The emphasis in belly breathing is on the exhalation, which can be extended by drawing in the abdominal muscles.

Belly breathing is great for relaxing at night, and I have taught it to many people who have difficulty with sleep. Lying down on your back put one hand on your belly; breathing in, your hand goes gently up, and breathing out it goes gently down. Breathing like this can help sleep because it has a physically relaxing effect (by switching on the rest and relax response) and because it gives the mind a gentle focus — many people have trouble sleeping because their minds are racing or churning over worries, so this helps to shift out of the talking and thinking mode into gentle body-awareness sensing mode.

DIAPHRAGMATIC BREATHING

The diaphragm is designed to be the main muscle involved in breathing, although it is supported by many others. Most of us have never been taught how to breathe, and many people often get into habits of using all the other muscles more than the diaphragm. This can lead to chronic tensions.

To breathe diaphragmatically, focus on using the diaphragm to breathe in. Imagine breathing more to the back of the body than the front, as there is more movement in the diaphragm there. Notice the lowest ribs expanding in your back. As the breath progresses the abdomen has a slight (but not exaggerated) movement forward, then the chest will expand a bit as the lower lungs fill and the breath fills upwards.

The muscles are active on the inhalation as the diaphragm pulls down and thickens. The diaphragm relaxes on the exhalation and naturally ascends back up, but the exhalation can also be supported by using the abdominal muscles, which can pull in, extending the exhale. When people are anxious they tend not to exhale very much, so focusing on the exhalation helps.

Once you have read the instructions above simply try to feel the diaphragm working — mostly the body knows how to do this, so just focusing on breathing using the diaphragm can often be enough. And remember that 'belly breathing' is another way to get much the same effect.

DIAPHRAGMATIC BREATHING WITH EXTENDED EXHALATION

Extending the exhalation increases the calm response (through the links to the vagus nerve — see pp. 46–47).

In this breath, the inhalation is through the diaphragm contracting, drawing the lungs down and the lower ribs out. The exhalation begins by just relaxing, so the diaphragm draws back in and up, then the muscles of the abdomen are used to squeeze in the belly (mostly the rectus abdominus at the front of the belly, but also the muscles on the sides). This lengthens the exhalation. Initially, focus on squeezing in these belly muscles, and then extend the squeezing by feeling that even the pelvic muscles pull in and up a little. While the pelvic muscles seem a long way from the lungs, incorporating them has a flow-on effect to make the exhalation longer.

This extension of the out-breath really turns on the 'calm switch' and once practised a little, even a single breath with a long, slow exhalation can produce a sense of calm. If you have any difficulty getting used to diaphragmatic breathing, focus initially on extending the exhalation by squeezing in the abdominal muscles — gently put your hand on your belly and push in as an aid to focus pulling in the belly. To get the feeling, you might imagine you are about to zip up a pair of jeans that are too tight.

THE FULL BREATH

One of the multitudes of different styles of breathing in yoga is so widely used that it is often called the 'yoga breath'.

The breath here is directed not just to the lower lungs, but to all the lung area.

It can be helpful to consider the lungs as divided into lower, middle and upper sections. Breathing into the lower part of the lungs is controlled by the diaphragm. Breathing into the middle part of the lungs is mostly controlled by the intercostal muscles, the muscles between the ribs. Breathing into the very top of the lungs is called clavicular breathing and can be controlled by using the muscles at the top of the chest, shoulders and neck.

The full breath involves breathing first into the lower lungs, contracting the diaphragm down (as in the diaphragmatic breathing on p. 65), then filling the middle part of the lungs by expanding the chest area, then filling the top of the lungs by widening the shoulders and opening out the top of the chest (make sure not to just lift up the shoulders and jam the neck; the shoulders stay broad). When breathing out, the breath is released first from the upper lungs, then the middle (contracting in the rib muscles), then the lower, letting the diaphragm ascend and pulling in the belly. [2]

Breathing this way floods the whole lungs with oxygen and has an energizing and rebalancing effect. This is an excellent breath to do for a few minutes each day as a regular practice. It has a very balanced effect, in that the breath to the higher part of the lungs stimulates the activation reflex, while breathing using the diaphragm stimulates the calm response — so the effect is that you feel alert but relaxed, which is ideal for most activities of the day.

While it is good to mostly practise the full breath in a slow and gentle manner, which has a balancing and calming effect, you can also practise it in a stronger, more muscular manner, which gives a feeling of strength and vitality. If you do it more strongly, a few breaths is enough so that you don't overdo it.

As you practise this breath, feel the breath drawn more to the back of the body, filling up the lower, middle sections then coming forward a little into the front of the upper chest at the end. This is subtle, so don't worry too much to begin with, but if you breathe more to the front of the body it has a more emotional effect — you wouldn't deliberately do this unless seeking to release some emotion. Breathing towards the back of the body is more calming. For more information about the front and back of the body, see pp. 70–71

FULL BREATH WITH PASSIVE EXHALATION

The full breath (as described on p. 67) can be done with a passive exhalation or controlled exhalation. For a passive exhalation, just let go after a full inhalation and the exhalation will occur due to the natural elasticity of the lungs (taking them back to the resting shape). The rib muscles come back in and the diaphragmatic muscle fibres relax, allowing the diaphragm to float up as the muscle relaxes and extends (reducing the volume of the lungs, which causes the out-breath). Having a controlled inhalation and passive exhalation allows a sense of coming back to balance, and should feel gently stimulating and relaxing. If you practise this a few times you will find that the length of the exhalation varies from day to day, depending on what is going on for you emotionally and how stressed or relaxed you are.

Do not hold the breath when doing this breathing, but allow any small, natural pauses to comfortably occur at the end of either the inhalation or exhalation.

CIRCULAR BREATHING

A specific variation of the full breath with passive exhalation is circular breathing, in which there is a deliberate moving from in-breath to out-breath without any pause in between. It is a great breath for releasing tension or helping to move through and release emotional blocks.

Circular breathing forms the basis of several psychotherapeutic techniques. There has been a lot written about it, in mostly 'new age' contexts. Doing this breath while deliberately relaxing, such as when lying down, is a simple, powerful and very helpful style of breathing. It gives a feeling of gently flooding the body with energy and releasing any pent up feelings.

To start, take a full controlled inhalation and then allow the exhalation to be passive. There should be ideally no break between the inhale and exhale (nor between the exhalation and the inhalation). You can continue this pattern as long as feels comfortable. Breathe in and out through your nose. Breathing in and out through the mouth lets more air in, so is stronger in some respects but also less refined. If you need to breathe through the mouth for this breath, breathe both in and out through the mouth. At the end you should allow the breath to return to its own rhythm and just gently relax for a few moments.

If you do this style of breathing on a few different occasions, you will probably notice that the length of the exhale varies a lot at different times. The length of exhalation seems to vary with your emotional state, and the breath helps to bring back some balance.

When doing this just stay gentle, so as not to overbreathe. If you start to feel dizzy or uncomfortable in any way just let go and let the breath be passive, or take a pause after an exhalation.

FULL BREATH WITH (MOSTLY) PASSIVE INHALATION

Most western physiology books focus on having a controlled inhalation and passive exhalation, but in yoga traditions the emphasis can be reversed, so as to take a full exhalation and then (since nature abhors a vacuum) allowing the lungs to refill passively. The breath is not entirely passive, but feels effortless.

This tends to have a calming effect. It can be good as a prelude to meditation, or as a practice for dealing with anxiety, so you gain more control over the muscles used in the exhalation (remembering that when anxious, focusing on a long, controlled exhalation is very helpful).

Take a full breath in to start, then let go and passively let out as much air as will release, then squeeze in the front of the belly (rectus abdominus) then the sides of the abdomen (transverse abdominus and obliques) and gently squeeze in the lower chest (using the intercostals). Afterwards, relax and allow the air to re-enter, gently drawing the dia-phragm down and out (so it is not entirely passive but feels effortless, like the floating of a jellyfish).

FULL BREATH WITH EXTENDED EXHALATION

The full breath can be extended by engaging the muscles of the belly to extend the exhalation. Breathe to the lower, middle and upper parts (as described on p. 67), then relax at the start of the exhalation; then as the upper and middle chest draw back in, squeeze in the muscles of the belly to squeeze out more of the air. This can be extended further by also drawing in and up the muscles at the base of the pelvis at the end. Although it might seem that these muscles are unrelated, you can feel the exhalation extend as you engage them — this has the benefit of strengthening the lower body and posture. When you breathe in again, gently release the abdominal muscles, but don't push the belly out. The muscles around the belly are passive on the inhalation.

Extending the exhalation has a calming effect, so that, combined with the full breath, it produces a meditative quality by being alert but relaxed.

BREATHING TO THE BACK OF THE BODY

You can direct a full breath down the back of the body, as if filling the body with breath from the base of the spine up the back of the body and finishing at the upper chest. Then reverse the breath to breathe out down the back of the body. Although the feelings are subtle, you can feel the back ribs spreading out as you do this, while the front of the chest stays relatively still. This style of breathing is calming and excellent as a prelude to meditation.

The notion that breathing to the back of the body should be calming sounds odd from a Western perspective, but generally in yoga and the Chinese practices of *chi kung* (also known as *qi gong*) the energy channels linked with the back of the body are calming while those linked with the front are energizing. Thus in the physical practice of yoga, doing backbends (opening the front of the body) is energizing, while forward bends (stretching the back) are calming.

To get used to the feeling of breathing to the back of the body a helpful practice is to sit in a chair and bend forward so that the body is forward over the thighs. This compresses the front of the body (making it difficult to breathe there) and opens the back. As you breathe you can feel the back ribs open out while the front ribs move very little. Breathing to the back becomes easier in this position and develops awareness of directing the breath to the back. Do a few breaths this way, then sit up straight and tall and continue breathing, doing full breaths while directing the breath to the back of the body. Imagine the breath going down to the base of the spine and filling up from the base of the spine, up the back of the body all the way to the top of the chest.

BPM

As well as where you direct the breath, another important focus is the length of the breath — how many breaths per minute (BPM).

There are simple but very important natural processes of the breath that just don't work properly if your rate of breathing is too fast. As we breathe in and the lungs expand, the change of pressure lets blood flow into the lungs, and as we breathe out blood flows out, so the flow of blood is supported beyond just relying on the pumping of the heart. As we breathe in the sympathetic nervous system (activation) is more engaged and as we breathe out the parasympathetic (calm response) is more activated. This relaxing response is largely due to the activation of the vagus nerve, but if the breath is too fast there is no real chance for this vagal activation to happen — the vagal brake (see pp. 46-47) is not activated and the system stays in sympathetic mode (fight or flight mode, i.e. stress). Breathing too fast or breathing in, holding the breath and only having a shallow exhalation acts to keep the body in stress mode.

Generally, slow breathing is good for you and the target zone is about five or six breaths per minute, or about five or six seconds in and five or six seconds out.[3] The idea is that this rate of breathing produces ideal sympathetic–parasympathetic balance and consistent, even heart rate variability. As we find this balance the body releases tensions, stress and anxiety and moves to ease, comfort and a sense of harmony.

Whether the exact optimum rate is five or six breaths differs with different research, and will vary a little from person to person in any case. Stephen Elliott, in his book *The New Science of the Breath*, insists that the ideal rate is 0.085 cycles per second (but I find this a bit hard to count, so five per minute is close enough). He argues that 'because the autonomic nervous system understands this frequency to be that of balance and ideal homeostasis, the heart rate variability rhythm will change to align with this breathing rhythm'. Elliott provides technical evidence to support this and examples of it helping people with problems including anxiety, anger management, pain, hypertension and addiction.[4]

Doctors Richard Brown and Patricia Gerbarg describe using this type of breathing with a range of people with dramatic results — including helping large groups of genocide trauma survivors in Rwanda and violence in Sudan.[5]

A range of evidence states that slower breathing is better, and that there is a 'sweet spot' in the rate of breathing that produces calm and balance and is ideal for healing.[6]

BREATHS PER MINUTE

If in trying this you find five or six breaths per minute a little slow for you, just slow the breath to whatever rate feels most comfortable. If seven or eight breaths per minute feels right for you, do that, and then after a week or two of practice, when you are used to it, experiment with slowing it a bit more. Some readers may be comfortable going even slower, but slower is probably more for meditation, so see how it feels for you to do five or six breaths per minute.

The basic technique is very much that of the full breath (see p. 67). To get the pace you might like to have a watch with a second hand, or just practise counting at about one count per second. The inhalation is active and the exhalation is passive. Allow the out-breath to be relaxed and passive, just letting the natural elasticity of the lungs gently expel the air. Breathe in and out through the nose. As you breathe in, be conscious to gently engage the diaphragm and then allow the middle and upper chest to also engage. Count or check a clock so that the inhalation is five or six seconds. Don't hold the breath, just exhale straight away or with a small, natural pause. Don't overbreathe — there should be no strain and plenty of 'reserve', so just do what feels comfortable and natural. If five seconds is too long, to begin with just breathe in and out for as long as is comfortable, keeping the same ratio (say, in for four and out for four).

Continue for several breaths, several minutes or however long suits you. Then just let go and let the breath become passive and notice how you feel.

SIMPLE MEDITATIVE BREATH

One of the best breathing styles for meditation, or simply to feel calm and peaceful, is to gently allow the breath to stream down the back of the body and then exhale up the front of body, completing a loop. This breath is gentle, feeling as if you allow it to happen rather than make it happen.

purposeful breathing

Sit on a chair with your back straight. In a natural 'straight' back there is a slight curving in of the lower spine — allow that natural curve. Sit forward on the edge of the chair, with your feet on the floor directly below your knees. Your back should not touch the back of the chair (when people do this they almost always slump). If you need the extra support of the back of the chair, use a cushion in your lower back to keep the natural curve of the lower back while sitting tall. Notice where the weight is on your sitting bones — if you rock slightly back or forward you can notice that the weight goes more to the back or front of the sitting bones. You want the weight to be just slightly forward, so there is a slight anterior (forward) tilt of the pelvis. Try to find the balance so that sitting feels relatively effortless. Breath education trainer Tess Graham suggests imagining a coathanger, as if your head and shoulders are the coathanger and everything else hangs gently from there.[7]

Gently begin breathing through the nose so that the breath goes to the back of the upper chest and then down the back of the chest, ultimately down the back ribs until the back portion of the diaphragm goes down — it should feel as if the breath is flowing down inside of the back ribs, almost to the pelvis. Then feel the breath complete a circuit as the exhalation rises up the front of the body. For the first few breaths you might control the exhalation, gently squeezing in at the belly and lower ribs, but after a few breaths try to allow this movement to happen as if of its own accord.

The breath should be gentle — allow the body to find the right amount of air coming in and out— and effortless. Don't ty to control the amount of the breath, just let it find its own balance. Allow the mind to be still and empty (this is often hard as the mind may jump, but this style of breathing helps to find this quietness — if your mind is jumpy you may want to do a more controlled style of breathing first). Just allow the breath to flow in through the nose, then down the back of the body, then out flowing up the front of the body, completing a loop.

Remember, the best breathing is about balance, not trying to breathe too much. In this style of breathing, just allow the body to direct how much is enough.

The beauty of this breath is its gentleness, which leads to a calm meditative state, as you let go and allow it to happen. It is no exaggeration to say that it often has a blissful quality.

RATIO BREATHING 1:2

Most of the main breathing styles in this book keep to the simple process of the in-breath and the out-breath at about the same length. There are times, though, when it is helpful to have a deliberately longer exhalation or inhalation. Extending the exhalation has a simple and profound calming effect, so is especially helpful when you are anxious, as the long exhalation triggers the relaxation response. A single long, slow exhale can definitely 'flick the calm switch' to help shift you out of a panicked state.

To extend the exhalation, relax after you have inhaled so that the exhale begins from the natural elasticity of the lungs. Then actively engage the muscles of the belly to squeeze in. The main muscles used are the rectus abdominus and the transverse abdominus. As suggested on p. 66, you can imagine pulling your belly in to fit into a tight pair of jeans. The end of the exhalation is further extended by drawing the pelvic muscles in and up.

A particular yoga breathing style is to breathe in and out to the ratio of one to two — so if you breathe in for a count of four then breathe out for a count of eight. This helps develop control of the muscles involved in breathing, enabling you to breathe fully, but the long exhalation also makes sure there is no overbreathing as its length helps balance the carbon dioxide levels. It also helps the parasympathetic nervous system response for calming the mind, so that there is sense of alert relaxation — excellent for meditation or for general health and healing.

To practise this breath, sit comfortably on a chair with your back straight, with the sitting bones on the front edge of the chair so you are not leaning back (which can cause slumping, and restricts the breath). Sit so the spine is long and naturally curves in a little in the lower back. Take a full breath in — imagine the breath going down the back of the body so you are filling up from the base of the back ribs, then filling up the middle, then chest and ending by filling up the upper chest. Always do this within comfortable limits; there should be no strain. Exhale by initially just relaxing so that the breath begins to exhale due to the elasticity of the lungs; then consciously draw in the muscles around the abdomen to squeeze the breath out, pulling them in, and at the end pull the muscles at the base of the pelvis in and up a little, which will help extend the exhale further (to get the feeling of this you can feel that the perineum — the point at the very base of the pelvis between the genitals and anus — pulls in and up, and even the anus pulls in and up). At the end of the exhalation breathe in again without totally letting go of the abdominal and pelvic muscles — they will release slowly and naturally as needed, so better not to just 'dump' the hold. Do a few rounds of this so you are used to the motion of it, then begin to count so that the length of the exhalation is twice the length of the inhalation. If it uncomfortable to manage the 1:2 count, then just get used to the breath with an even count, or slowly progress towards the ratio, say by breathing in for four and then out for six. If you feel any discomfort, just stop and let the breath return to its own rhythm.

Breathing like this has the benefit of being good for posture, and helps bring life into the muscles that hold the 'core' of the body in place.

Breathing in ratio can be done the other way around, such that the inhalation is twice the length of the exhalation; this will have an energizing effect. Taking a longer inhalation and stronger, shorter exhalation might be helpful if you are drowsy and want to lift yourself a little, or could be used if you are exercising and wanting to get more oxygen to your muscles, breathing in then exhaling forcefully and more quickly. A few breaths like this is plenty, though, and it would not usually be done as a regular practice as it can quickly lead to overbreathing. By contrast, having the ratio of 1:2 inhalation to exhalation can be practised for prolonged periods.

BREATH HOLDING

Holding the breath is something many people do unconsciously. You might imagine having a shock, gasping in air and holding it. Sometimes people hold their breath in suspense.

Usually for breath holding we think of holding the breath in, but there can also be a stopping of breath after exhaling. Sometimes people caught in deeply sad thoughts sigh out, then have a long pause before breathing in again.

Holding the breath can be used to great advantage in yoga and meditative practices. Some breath holding is extraordinary, as in the increasingly popular sport of free diving. Diving deep in the ocean on a single breath has a beauty to it but also carries risks, so those doing it are usually well prepared and have trained extensively. Nonetheless it is something to be approached with caution. Holding the breath in will tend to raise your blood pressure, so is not good for anyone whose blood pressure is already high. If you try breath holding it should not be strenuous.

In yoga breathing, breath holding is done when you are already relaxed, so there is a conscious balance of effort and subtle awareness of effect.

One simple breath-holding method is the 4-7-11 breath — you breathe in for a count of four, hold for seven then exhale for a count of eleven. I personally don't recommend such a pattern, as it is complicated and runs a risk of harm as the person might strain to do it. Even in yoga, breath holding is usually only done after long periods of practising breathing *without* holding — so that there are very high levels of interoceptive awareness, noticing what is happening as you do it.

Generally, holding in the breath raises energy levels. Taking a full breath and briefly holding it can be a helpful pick-up if you are feeling drowsy. On the other hand, holding the breath out after an exhalation tends to lower energy levels. Done as part of a meditative practice, this has the effect of stilling the mind and bringing you into a state of quiescence. In daily life, holding the breath out for brief periods can be helpful if you have been overbreathing. It will raise carbon dioxide levels, which brings things back to balance if you tend to hyperventilate.

In general, though, holding the breath in or out should be done cautiously.

More on the nose and mouth

It is generally better to breathe through the nose. As well as humidifying and purifying the air, it allows a far greater awareness of controlling an even flow of air. With an open mouth it is very easy to dump or gasp in big bursts of air.

If your nose is blocked, however, a good alternative is to simply reduce the size of the opening of the mouth, so that the flow of air is reduced, which allows a slowing of the breath and more ability to make it even. One way to do this is to purse the lips and to imagine breathing in and out through a straw. The more even the breath, the more balanced your mental state.

Noticing the nostrils

As you pay more attention to the breath, you are likely to notice times when the passage of air flows more freely through one nostril or the other. This flow of air more through one nostril actually changes in rhythmic patterns through the day. These rhythms have long been known in yoga circles and have recently received attention in the West as 'ultradian' rhythms, linked with different styles of thought and mood, such as moving between focused, rational states or more associational daydreaming states.

Generally, we move between having one nostril freer (or more dominant in the flow) every 90 minutes or so, though the length of time may vary.

If you stop now and then to notice which nostril is predominant you will see this shift, with sometimes the flow of air through each nostril being fairly even as you are transferring from one to the other. You might like to notice now if one nostril is clearer than the other. You can gently press one side of your nose with a finger to breathe in and out from the opposite nostril, then change sides and notice which is easier and clearer. If you remember, check occasionally through the day and you will notice times when one nostril or the other is more open, and transition times when they are in balance.

In yoga, there are three main energy channels and many more minor ones. The main energy channels are *shushumna*, which travels up the spine, and *ida* and *pingala*, which interweave up and down the spine. *Ida* is linked with the left nostril and *pingala* with the right. *Ida* is a more cooling 'moon' energy and *pingala* a more fiery 'sun' energy. One of the yoga breathing practices is to breathe through alternate nostrils so as to balance these energies.

In the yoga tradition each nostril is linked with a different major energy channel of the body. As yoga has come to be been linked with more modern Western understandings, brain function has also been seen as connected to the nostrils. Breathing through the right nostril is thought to link with stimulating the left hemisphere of the brain, and the left nostril with the right hemisphere of the brain. Western psychology tells us that the left hemisphere is usually associated with language-based thinking and analytic skills, and the right with creative, associative and imagery-based thinking.

In the ancient traditions it was said that if you only breathed through one nostril for prolonged periods it created a sustained imbalance. There is even a claim in the poetic language of the time that if you breathed through one nostril only for four days, death would result — rather exaggerated, but it makes a clear point.

Western medical knowledge has recently discovered that depression is often linked with activity of the right frontal cortex of the brain. The right cortex is linked with general mood states, so may link with generalized negative thoughts (and, in fact, simple highly detailed tasks can be helpful for shifting out of general depressed moods — things like the now popular adult coloring books, because this activates the left cortex). Links of such prolonged mood states with nostrils are still being researched, but Amy Weinstraub, author of a book on using yoga to treat depression reports the case of a man who had a deviated right septum and hence could not breathe fully through his right nostril. Breathing through his left nostril meant he stimulated only the right hemisphere, the 'creative, artistic, non-verbal side of his brain' and she suggests this was linked with his depression. 'To compensate for his still-deviated right septum,' says Weinstraub, 'he began a regular practice of Right-Nostril breathing, also known as Vitality-Stimulating Breath (*Surya Bheda*). He reported that "twenty years of depression lifted like a cloud". Weinstraub also notes, 'He had also given up drinking and had Western psychotherapy, but he felt the breathing was "the crowning touch".[8]

The effects of prolonged breathing through one or the other nostril are not clearly established in Western research, but it does seem clear that breathing through the nostrils in an alternate and balanced fashion leads to a balancing of energies and also of brain activity.[9]

ALTERNATE NOSTRIL BREATHING

In the yoga tradition this alternate nostril breathing is called *nadi sodhana* (or energy channel cleansing). One teacher, Rama Jyoti Vernon, says *nadi sodhana* is an excellent balancing practice, and that whether a student has 'too much fire' (anxiety or mania) or 'not enough' (dysthymia, major depression), breathing in this way 'neutralizes the energy'.[10]

Deliberately breathing for a period of time through only one nostril purposely creates an imbalance so is best done only under expert guidance. By contrast, the practice of breathing through alternate nostrils is safe and widely used. In this practice, you use the thumb and fingers of the right hand to block each nostril alternately. It is traditional to curl the index and middle fingers of the right hand in to the palm of the hand, using the ring and little finger to block one nostril and the thumb to block the other. If this feels too awkward, you can use the thumb and the index finger to press on either side of the nose.

Begin by gently pressing the thumb just under the bony part halfway up the nose on the right side, while you breathe in through the left nostril; then release the thumb, and gently block the left nostril, pushing the ring and little finger against the left nostril just under the bony part; then breathe out through the right nostril; then breathe in through the right nostril; then change the fingers and breathe out through the left nostril. This completes one cycle. Do several cycles. Put more briefly, one cycle is:

breathe in through the left nostril
breathe out through the right nostril
breathe in through the right nostril
breathe out through the left nostril.
Keep the breath gentle and breathe slowly.

If you do this for several minutes (three to five or more) it brings a sense of clarity, lightness and balance. If one of your nostrils is blocked, you can either wait until it clears and come back to the practice after half an hour or so, or lie on your side for a few moments; with the blocked side uppermost, the nasal congestion usually clears as the gunk gets moved by gravity, or place the hand of the blocked side under the armpit of the opposite arm, press up gently and squeeze for a few minutes (an old yoga trick which clears the opposite nostril).

Alternate nostril breathing is a great breath for feeling relaxed, alert and focused. It's therefore perfect when taking a break from, or just before starting, office work or study. When I use it, I find it helps my creative and logical thinking work well together. It is also excellent before meditation. It is also a great breath for bringing things back into balance. If you find your mind is churning over things and it is hard to switch off, or that you are stuck in a general down mood, alternate nostril breathing shifts you out of these states to bring a sense of peaceful balance.

Any conscious breath

While there are quite a number of different styles of breathing listed in this book, one of the most important points is that *any breath* can be helpful in feeling calmer, stronger and more centred, as long as it is conscious and relatively slow. If you feel at all confused by some of the breathing styles, then forget the detail for a while and just take a slow breath with awareness. Don't worry about how slow; just make sure it is not racing.

Any slow breath with awareness will help to calm you. This is partly because when people feel stressed or anxious they are usually thinking stressed or anxious thoughts, and just pausing to focus on the breath for a moment helps to shift out of the racing thoughts and into simple body awareness — out of that self-talk mode into sensing mode. This is calming, and gives you a pause with which to centre yourself, and to step a little out of the flow of thoughts to decide how best to relate to whatever is happening. Secondly, any slower breath gives a chance for the calming system to kick in, and to shift out of fight or flight, or stress, mode. A few slow, conscious breaths helps to bring everything back into more balance, making you a little calmer and more centred.

So if some of the anatomical bits seem awkward or take a while to master, just practise taking any slow conscious breath. Then as you practise, work gently on making the breath deep rather than high. That's enough, you don't have to work through all the details.

Just keep breathing

It may sound a bit dumb to say it, but often the most important thing to do is just keep breathing. In many emotional situations it is a natural response to hold our breath. There are a few times when this can be helpful, such as providing a moment's pause in situations of threat, and sometimes you may want to contain your emotions a little. Occasionally this is helpful as you might want to 'take a deep breath and just do it'. Most of the time, however, it makes it more difficult to respond fluidly to the situation at hand. In a counselling context I often notice people stop breathing (either literally stopping or greatly restricting their breathing) when they are dealing with a difficult emotion. The encouragement to 'just keep breathing' is very helpful for processing and releasing through the emotion. Generally, just keeping breathing (that is, not holding the breath or having much of a break between the inhalation and the exhalation) allows the emotion to move through.

This breath restriction can be part of many psychological problems. Psychologist Stephen Wolinsky makes the point that many psychological problems are linked with a narrowing of attention, like a hypnotic trance state — when someone is highly depressed or anxious they operate in a restricted way, being stuck in their thoughts and emotions, unable to access resources that might otherwise be available.[11] He notes that this typically happens with a holding of the breath. The person holds the breath and becomes caught in this negative trance state. Of course, this happens unconsciously, but if they *just keep breathing slowly and deeply* they also begin to shift out of this problematic state.

Remembering to just keep breathing generally leads to a breath that fits the moment, something which is both helpful and enjoyable. When we are conscious of breathing it is more likely to be slow and full. Conscious breathing in this fashion is one of the small, subtle pleasures of life, as the breath can be enjoyed and used to enhance the moment.

Breathing with awareness

While this chapter has described specific styles of breathing, a key focus is the development of more personal awareness. Each individual's styles of breathing might vary markedly. You might like to simply stop and notice your breath every now and then. Just notice where the air goes (such as deep or high in the lungs), how fast or slow, and how shallow or deep the breath is. If you become more aware of your own breathing patterns, you'll also become more aware of when you may want to purposefully direct the breath in a number of ways for relaxing, recharging or to otherwise change mood or state of mind.

While most of the focus of this book is on developing awareness of your own breathing, it can also help to notice the breathing of others around you. It may be a bit weird if you start staring at people's chests, but watching TV is a simple way to develop awareness of breathing patterns. Look at how the actors breathe and how this changes with different emotional, physical and mental states. Once you start tuning in to this, you will see endless examples. A favourite example of mine for a good use of high breathing can be seen on the TV series *The Borgias*. In this series, Jeremy Irons plays the pope at around the year 1500. Surrounded by cardinals and intrigue, he plots and wields power. There are several moments in the series in which Irons, as the Borgia pope, acts to make a decision and issue an imperious edict. At these moments he breathes forcefully and fully through the nostrils, and high into the chest — filling the upper chest fully (not the high gasp of the frightened) — there is a sense of command with this breath, of assuming the role of ruler, of being above the fray. He captures it perfectly.

Another example is Sylvester Stallone in the old *Rocky* series. When struggling with titanic effort, he sucks down air. His mouth is open, always a little to one side, and there is a powerful pull of deep diaphragmatic breathing. You can feel, even on the screen, that there is a real physical power to it.

Breath snacks

The more you focus on breathing, the more you can become aware of it as a simple source of joy. Even a single breath, when given our full attention, is a powerful reminder that we are alive, and what a remarkable thing that is. It directs attention to the drawing in of life energy. It allows our physicality to be felt as an active thing, interlinked with emotions and ways of thinking.

Just stopping now and again and taking a few purposeful breaths feels good, grounds you in your body and, depending on the style of the breath, can be calming, centring or energizing. It is a definite snack right up there with coffee or biscuits, totally healthy and calorie free.

PART 3

Breathing for specific purposes

7

STOP, BREATHE, REFOCUS

This chapter describes specific breathing styles to use for specific purposes.

At the outset, however, it is important to remind yourself that almost any slow, conscious breath can be helpful to reset the system. Simply focusing on and controlling the breath helps to move out of the 'talking/thinking' modes that link with anxious thoughts, angry thoughts or depressive ruminations. Moving into a 'sensing, body-awareness mode' in itself interrupts unhelpful thought patterns. Once you step out of the thought loops and have a moment of mental quietness and calm, you can refocus.

Of course, this is not totally new. Maybe when you were a child your grandparents told you to 'take a deep breath and count to ten'. If you were very angry and then held your breath for a count of ten, you might have been at risk of bursting a blood vessel, but the idea of a deep breath interrupting agitation was there. And maybe your grandparents braced themselves before a challenge with a deep breath, or pumped themselves up with a few strong breaths. So on the one hand it is nothing new, but on the other hand we can refine and expand the practice to make it more effective, more powerful and more accessible.

As a general practice, two all-purpose breaths are diaphragmatic breathing for shifting out of any anxiety state (see p. 65) or the 'full breath' for most everything else (see p. 67). This 'full' breath has a calming effect due to the slowness and diaphragmatic involvement, but is also activating as it is full and breathes into the upper chest.

Shifting gears

The simple phrase 'Stop, breathe, refocus' is a helpful guide to shifting gears in stressful situations. Just stop, take three or four breaths — such as the full breath — and then refocus. This refocusing can then be with a view to the state you want to be in — to be calm, for example, or task directed.

While this is deliberately very simple, it is not always obvious how to refocus or what to refocus on. The refocusing can be guided by one or other of three levels: your immediate task, your bigger goals or your most important values. Sometimes one or other of them will be the most important thing in refocusing.

- **Task.** The task is the immediate thing you are trying to achieve. If you are studying or working at a desk and you find yourself becoming tired, distracted or anxious about completing your task, then you can stop, take a few deep breaths, and remind yourself of your immediate task — which may be to complete a paragraph of writing or piece of work. The specific breathing styles can be to energize, calm or centre. If you have been studying for a while you may need a break, but otherwise the task is to 'refocus' on completing that page, or that section — that is, to stop, breathe and refocus on the task at hand. This is simple and perhaps a bit obvious in theory, but very helpful in practice. If it is a long task, then having simple phrases to say, like 'one step at a time', can help.
- **Goals** are broader and may be short-term or long-term.

Typical goals might be achieving key performance indicators at work, completing a degree, meeting sales targets, buying a car or a house or having a great vacation after a period of work. If you are bored, anxious, panicked or depressed while doing an activity then it can help to stop, breathe and refocus on the goal. If you are anxious about giving a talk, reminding yourself of the goal may help (whatever that is for you: raising support for a cause, completing requirements for work or study). Having clear goals helps, of course. The breathing can help shift mood or emotional state and then you can refocus on the goal.

- **Values** are different and perhaps even more important though less obvious. Values are ways of being that you want to live by; qualities you want to have more fully in your life; character strengths; principles; or standards of behaviour. Aligning with our core values gives direction to life in ways that are satisfying, rewarding and fulfilling. An example might be that you want to be loving and loved, show courage, be creative or fair. These values are something we live with and can live by, so there is no particular end to them, in contrast to a goal that can be achieved and then is done. For example, if your goal is to get married, once you are married the goal is achieved, so you need a new goal (maybe you can get a quick divorce so you can get married again). On the other hand, if your value is to have a life filled with love, then marriage may be a step on the path, with ongoing opportunities to give and receive love, deepen the relationship and so on.

More on values

There can be many of these values, but one classification has been put forward by psychologists Christopher Peterson and Martin Seligman.[1] They speak of character strengths that they suggest are universal, present in all cultures and that represent values in action.

Peterson and Seligman cluster 24 key values in action under six broader categories:

1. **Wisdom and knowledge: values of creativity, curiosity, sound judgement, love of learning and clear perspective.**
2. **Courage: having bravery, perseverance, honesty and zest for life.**
3. **Humanity: having love, kindness and social intelligence.**
4. **Justice: valuing teamwork, fairness and leadership.**
5. **Temperance: valuing forgiveness, humility, prudence and self-regulation.**
6. **Transcendence: gratitude, hope, humour, spirituality and having an appreciation of beauty.** [2]

Although this list of values has a lot of research behind it, it is not an absolute list. You could think of other values, related to or distinct from those above, such as authenticity, balance, recognition, fame, friendships, loyalty, optimism, self-respect, trustworthiness, wealth or wisdom.

What can really help with resetting your system is to be able to remind yourself of what your top two or three values are. If you are doing a task that is highly stressful, for example, then reminding yourself of your key values will help align you with the task and channel the stress into productivity. If the task is not worth doing then perhaps don't do it, but the nature of doing the task changes when you feel it aligns with your values — whether that be helping others, or a love of learning, fairness, loyalty or being artistic. The breathing allows a way to interrupt problem states like anxiety or boredom and reset your mind in line with these values.

DEFINING YOUR VALUES

Take a moment to think of what your main three values are at this moment in your life. Use the lists above as a start, but feel free to add any other values that come to mind.

As an example, say the three most important values for you are to love and be loved, develop and deepen friendships, and succeed at your career. So if you were to stop, breathe and refocus, you might remind yourself of 'love, friendship and success'. Or perhaps for you it may be spirituality, gratitude and loyalty. Or fairness, leadership and wisdom.

Having more than three is okay, of course, but two or three are easy to remember and easy to remind yourself of at times of stress.

The three values I often use as a guide for myself are integrity, love and humour. This is not to say that I embody these virtues, nor even to suggest that I am any good at them. But if I align myself with these then I feel more energized and at peace with myself. Self-doubts, self-criticism and anxieties tend to diminish. If I act with integrity in the sense of acting with honesty and good intentions, then I can feel secure in my work and know I can sleep at night. Acting with love in the broad sense of caring for others, like Christian love or Buddhist loving-kindness, just feels better, hopefully helps others, in a small way helps to make the world a bit better and is more likely, most of the time, to build better relationships. Humour is not always appropriate but it can also have the broader meaning of 'good humour' and I always look for humour with warmth — all of us share our human faults and frailties, all of us are half ape and half angel, and sharing some humour invites us to share the human condition together. If humour is not appropriate, then warmth is fine. The point here is that if I feel stressed or threatened, reminding myself of these values helps me feel better and be more productive. This also produces a physical change (as will be discussed on p. 103), in that aligning with your values turns the biology of stress into the biology of courage: more good brain chemicals are released, blood vessels are less constricted and there is a greater sense of connection. So if I feel stressed or anxious I often stop, breathe and refocus. Sometimes the refocusing is just on the task if I have been distracted, but often it is on the bigger picture.

Breathing for calm

CALMING WITH A SINGLE BREATH

The best single way to help rapidly calm yourself is to take a long exhalation. Breathing in and out through the nose is usually best but you can also breathe out through pursed lips, as if breathing out through a straw. You might like to practise this now: take in a breath and then form a small round hole with pursed lips, as if you had a straw through which you are breathing; then breath out slowly, letting the narrowness of the opening control the rate of the exhalation. The long, slow exhalation activates the vagus nerve, so physically changes the system to a more relaxed mode, switching on the calming response.

If you think of the 1 to 10 scale (in which 1 is completely relaxed and 10 is totally stressed) a single breath won't take you from 10 to 0, but will usually take you down at least a couple of notches, such as from 7 to a 5 or 4.

CALMING IN A FEW BREATHS

When breathing to bring calm, the emphasis is always on the exhalation. The diaphragmatic breathing with extended exhalation on p. 66 is typically the best breath to use to find a sense of calm. If you have not practised it then the easiest thing to do to calm yourself is the 'belly' breath, breathing as if to the belly. More specifically, make sure you are mostly using the diaphragm. Putting your hand on your belly helps focus attention there, and then squeeze in the abdominal muscles to extend the exhalation. A simple focus is that breathing in, the belly goes out, and breathing out, the belly goes in.

Then slow it down, ideally to about five seconds in and five or more seconds out.

Ray

Ray saw me for help because he was very stressed and agitated, and was becoming overwhelmed. He had an important meeting coming up and felt he would make a disaster of it. I noticed in the session that he breathed both high in the chest and through his mouth. I explained that a different style of breathing may help and he agreed to try.

When people are very agitated or anxious, focusing on the belly is easier to grasp than focusing on the diaphragm. I did the breathing with him and he began to slow his breath down. I modelled the action by having one hand on my own belly and with the other I pointed with my index finger, placing it on the hand on the belly, and emphasized squeezing in on the out-breath. I had him place his hand on his belly so he could gently push in on the exhalation to help draw focus to the abdominal muscles. Over the course of a few breaths he could extend the exhalation. I then gently added a slow count to help him be aware of slowing the breath and making it more even. We did another three or four of these breaths then I told him to relax and let go of the breath. In all we had done about nine or ten breaths. I asked about his anxiety on the scale of 0 to 10 and he had gone from 8.5 to 5. When I asked how he felt now, he said 'calmer'.

During the rest of the session we looked at other factors including anxious thoughts and how to manage them, strengths he could build upon, and ways to constructively prepare for the meeting, and before the end of the session we came back to practise the breathing again to consolidate it. He said he was happy to practise the breath, as are most people because the difference is so immediate.

THE SLOW LEAK

This breath is a simple option for switching on the calm response for anyone having difficulty with diaphragmatic breathing. It allows a slow, gentle exhalation.

Breathe in slowly and fully, in whatever way is available for you, preferably through the nose. Then, purse the lips as if you are about to breathe out through a very small straw (another way to think of this is to purse the lips as if you are about to whistle). Make the hole created by the lips as small as you can. Then relax and let the breath seep out as if the hole is allowing a slow leak of the air. With this breath it is important not to push the breath out, as the pressure against the small aperture would create tension. It should feel relaxed, like slowly letting air out of a balloon. When the breath out has finished, breathe in slowly again and repeat.

One benefit of this breath is that it is available to almost anyone, and the slowness of the exhale allows the calming response. With this breath it is easy to be able to have the exhalation be at least five seconds, and often eight or ten seconds is comfortable.

Evie

Evie saw me for help with a range of stresses, including working through past traumas and current work stress. She had several health problems, including a quite severe gastro-intestinal problem that meant she had to have a very restricted diet. She was also seeing a doctor and naturopath. She had recently had a period of intense illness in which she was exhausted and spent several days in bed. She had had episodes like this at times in the past.

As we explored Evie's situation, it seemed that one of the issues was when she became very stressed it was very hard for her to shift out of the stress state; she would stay on edge and her mind would race from one worry to the next. This sustained stress state had a very negative impact on her immune system, which was then weakened and other underlying health problems overwhelmed her. At these times, other health-maintaining activities that she did, such a going for walks, became too hard and unavailable. As we talked, her breath was high in the chest, often held, and her exhalation was often quite quick and shallow.

Although only one part of treatment, it seemed that controlled breathing could help Evie by allowing her to switch off the stress response and switch on the calming response, which would help her body to heal. When we began to do the breathing it was clear she could not really engage her diaphragm in deep breathing, as her abdominal area was painful and sensitive. The slow leak breath was a good option for her — she could breathe in slowly and as much as was comfortable for her, then just let the breath seep out through the small opening of her lips. This allowed her exhalation to slow to several seconds, and with that she began to feel calmer and more relaxed. She was able to practise this at home and it became part of her recovery, as she could more consciously enter the bodily rest and repair mode and feel more empowered that she could take some action, rather than just being victim to her condition.

EXTENDING THE SENSE OF CALM AND FOCUS

Another option for developing a general sense of calm is to breathe more to the back of the body than the front. This is a subtle but important shift.

One way to develop this breath is to sit in a chair and then bend forward, so your belly and chest are on or near your thighs, your head hanging down a little towards the floor. In this position you will feel that breathing to the front of body is constricted, and you can then direct the breath up the back. Try to inhale right to the base of the spine, then to the back of the abdomen and back of the chest, feeling the back ribs expand and finishing at the back of the shoulders, feeling the shoulder blades open out. Then exhale from the shoulders, down through the chest and all the way out from the lower back. Breathing like this begins to open the back more and develop awareness of breathing to the back.

Once you have this awareness you can just sit normally and direct the breath to the back, breathing all the way from the pelvis up to the shoulders and breathing out from the shoulders all the way down to the base of the spine.

From an Eastern perspective, different energy channels are stimulated if we breathe to the back than if we breathe to the front of the body. Also as you feel the breath go down the back, it draws the diaphragm down in a different way to breathing to the front of the body or breathing higher in the chest.

To sum up, the main principles of breathing for calm are:

- **Breathe deep as if to the belly** rather than high in the chest.
- **The slower the breath the more calming it is,** as long as it stays reasonably comfortable, of course (not so slow as to be forced or make you short of breath).
- **Don't hold the breath in** — however, pausing after the exhalation can sometimes be calming, especially if you have been overbreathing.
- **Extending the exhalation is calming.** The slower the exhalation the more calming the breath, as long as it is within comfortable limits.
- **Focusing on the breath in itself tends to help calm you because it helps redirect the mind.** When people are anxious, their anxious thoughts feed the anxiety further. Focusing on the breath tends to interrupt this as you go from a mode of self-talking to a mode of gentle body awareness.

8

MANAGING AND TRANSFORMING STRESS

One of the problems in the modern world is that we are often under stress for long periods. The system that is activated when we are stressed, the fight or flight system, is designed through evolution to only be activated for short periods, for escape or defence.

The bad news about stress can be found in countless magazines and newspaper articles as well as academic journals. The stress chemicals designed for brief bursts of activity are kicked off throughout the day. The main chemical of concern is cortisol. Cortisol helps release energy in the short-term, but long-term it is bad for the immune system among other things. Additionally, having adrenaline hanging around in the system also keeps us on edge.

Stress management strategies include exercise, because the body is geared for major activity when stressed. Doing any sort of cardio exercise will help to burn off and flush through the cortisol and adrenaline, and also releases a few endorphins, which help you feel calmer and happier.

Boosting performance: getting into 'the zone'

While prolonged stress is bad for us, some stress can be helpful.

A certain amount of stress can enhance performance, and the relation between stress and performance was first put forward more than 100 years ago, in 1908.[1] Known as the Yerkes-Dodson law and represented by an inverted U, it is helpful when considering performance at work or, say, for a student in exams. This law states that if there is too little stress the person might not really 'switch on' or not be motivated enough to perform at their best. Too much stress, on the other hand, and performance starts to be impacted and diminish. Recognizing this means that you can get more into your own 'optimal zone' for performing at your best. If you go into the too-high zone you can use breathing to help you return to the optimal performance zone. Deep diaphragmatic breathing can help here (see p. 65), as when most people get stressed and anxious the breath becomes high in the chest, and diaphragmatic breathing shifts that. The full breath (p. 67) is another option — drawing the breath deep and to the back will enhance the calming and centring effect.

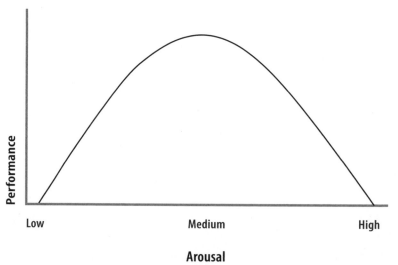

Arousal

('Arousal' here meaning physiological arousal, especially stress or anxiety.)

Rethinking stress: some good news

More generally, how we approach stress makes a huge difference. Recent research has also shown many positive associations with stress, and that it seems we have several different stress responses, not just the fight or flight response.

Health psychologist Kelly McGonigal has drawn together a range of this research to show how stress can be used productively. One very interesting study was conducted with 30,000 American adults. They were followed up over an eight-year period to see what effects different levels of stress had upon their health. After eight years it was found that those with high levels of stress had a 43 per cent increased risk of dying, *but only those who had high stress and believed that it was bad for them.* Those who had high stress but did not see it as harmful had lower risk of death, even lower than those who experienced little stress.[2]

It seems that how we view stress has a lot of key physiological effects. If people view stress as harmful, their blood vessels constrict, raising blood pressure. When they view it as helpful, the blood vessels stay open, so more blood is pumped and oxygenated, which helps better performance.

Stress and the good hormones

Stress triggers the release of a number of hormones as well as adrenaline and cortisol. Oxytocin is also released. Oxytocin has a physical effect of helping to repair the heart, and is linked with connections with other people, such as hugging and breastfeeding. It is often called the 'cuddle hormone'. Often people will think of stress as making them withdraw or be more competitive with others, but a number of studies now show that mostly stress gears people to look after those close to them, reach out for help and want to support others. This has been referred to as the 'tend and befriend' response. Imagine a parent protecting their children at a time of danger, or the way that so many people reach out to help others in threatening situations. Recognizing this can help, because we can seek help and support others when stressed.

The other stress chemical that is released is DHEA (dehydroepiandros-terone). DHEA is a brain steroid. It enhances specific learning so that you can potentially learn better when stressed. It also speeds up wound repair and enhances immune function, offsetting some of the damage of cortisol.

Some studies have looked at levels of cortisol and DHEA released in stressful situations. High levels of cortisol are associated with impaired immune function and depression. High levels of DHEA, however, are asso-ciated with *reduced* risk of anxiety, depression, heart disease, neurodegen-eration and other stress related conditions.[3] The ratio of DHEA to cortisol is called the *growth index* of the stress response. A higher growth index — more DHEA compared to cortisol — is linked to thriving under stress.

Researcher Alia Crum had participants take part in a mock job inter-view in which interviewers were trained to make the situation deliberately stressful (giving lots of frowns, rolling their eyes, looking disapproving). There were two experimental groups: before the interview each participant was shown either a three-minute video outlining how stress was bad or how stress was enhancing (both videos were based on real research but selective in what they presented). At end of interview, saliva was taken from participants. Those who had seen the 'positive perception of stress' video had higher 'growth index' — a higher proportion of DHEA to cortisol. Perception of stress (in this instance, from simply watching a three-min-ute video) altered not just attitudes, but actual physiology in response, and more positive brain steroids were released.[4]

Getting more of the benefits

One way to use stress better is to think of it as gearing your body and brain to perform better. Before a big sports game most people will feel excited — 'pumped up' or 'stressed' in a positive way. Viewing stress before a work meeting or an exam can be much the same — it gears us to perform better and if we think of it that way, then all sorts of positive physiologi-cal responses flow from that (more brain steroids, better blood flow to the brain etc.).

It also helps to recognize that a lot of the original research on the negative effects of stress was done on animals who were (let's face it, some early psychology experiments were pretty horrible) stressed physically to near the point of death. Some of our stress responses might be like that — if we are in a war or a car crash, or assaulted — but many stress situations are milder and different in nature. This is not to suggest that all stress is positive, but the new research does suggest that there are ways to get the best or worst out of each situation and that some stress can be positive.

One of the best ways to harness the best of stress is to ask how what we are doing can be linked to meaningful goals. If you are studying to get the career you want in order to help others, contribute to making the world a better place or even just to make lots of cash, then reminding yourself of what is meaningful for you and how the stressful situations allow you to move closer to achieving those goals, will help to perform better, learn better and get the best out of the stressful situation.

So when you feel stressed, it can help to use the 'stop, breathe, refocus' technique described on p. 90. This simple act can shift the task so it feels more like a challenge, something worthwhile. With this simple shift there is a physiological shift as well; blood vessels contract less and the positive hormones kick in.

If you are really stressed and it doesn't align with your core values, maybe it is better to stop and do something else, or to stop and see if there is a bigger picture, such as doing a job you don't like but doing it to provide for the family you love.

It does make a real difference if we can align ourselves to goals that are bigger than we are. Helping other people, working towards bigger goals and connecting with others all help to transform stress into a source of energy.

Breathing to 'centre', boost willpower and determination

To say someone 'feels centred' implies a sense of feeling calm and self-assured. It also implies a physical sense of being strong and graceful, and is the opposite of being 'scattered' or 'unbalanced'.

When you feel distracted or caught up in powerful emotions, it can be very helpful to find a feeling of being centred. Focusing on the breath provides a simple way of doing that, using the 'stop, breathe, refocus' strategy (see p. 90).

If you are feeling agitated one simple way to help calm yourself is to do deep diaphragmatic breathing (p. 65). The full breath (p. 67) is also excellent for centring.

Having taken a few breaths, remind yourself of your goals, ideals or key values, which allows a refocus and reinvigoration. And it helps, too, to remember that channelling the energy of the stress allows not just mental but also actual physiological changes linked with strength and courage.

HARA BREATH

One of the best breaths to both centre and boost energy is to breathe to the *hara*. This is the most common name for the energy centre located behind the navel (depending on your body shape, it is behind the navel or a few centimetres below the navel and in towards the centre of the body). The *hara* is located roughly at the body's centre of gravity. The same centre is known as the *tan tien* (or lower *tan tien*) in the Chinese energy systems and is linked with *manipura chakra* in yoga. In martial arts, being centred here gives balance. Stability and force are created as you operate out of your core.

For our purposes it is helpful to recognize that the *hara* is a very helpful place to direct the breath and your attention if you feel under threat or need to calm down, or are facing challenges for which you want to summon your willpower.

To breathe to the *hara*, imagine the breath being taken down the centre of the body, slightly towards the back of centre (but not down the front). From a Western perspective, the air we breathe does not literally go into the belly, but breathing as *if* it goes there affects the areas of the lungs to which the breath is drawn. Breathing as if to the belly draws the diaphragm down and the air goes deep into the lungs.

The breath should engage the diaphragm as you breathe in, and by imagining this you can activate more the back of the diaphragm, as if the breath was going to the *hara* point. The exhalation can be strengthened by pulling in the muscles of the belly so it is more forceful and has a muscular quality.

If you breathe strongly and forcefully to the *hara* point it has the effect of 'charging up' the body while allowing you to still keep a steady focus. It is the sort of breath a martial artist might use before trying to smash some bricks. It is energizing but allows a continuing feeling of 'being centred'. Usually you would just do this for a few breaths, as to pump the air too much like this can lead to overbreathing. So a few breaths are usually enough to charge you up while feeling centred. This is unlike rapid breathing high in the lungs, which leads people to 'spin out'.

This centring can be done gently and slowly to be calming, or more strongly to energize and aid strength and determination.

When you do the breath in a more muscular fashion, try to feel the back of the diaphragm working on the inhale and make sure to emphasize squeezing the muscles in on the exhale. Doing the breath in a more muscular fashion is helpful when you want to feel strong or forceful.

Breathing to release tension

The first step for releasing tension is to make sure you are not breathing in a way that creates it — high breathing, rapid breathing or 'reverse' breathing are likely to make you tense and then keep you tense. Slow, deep diaphragmatic (p. 65) or full breathing (p. 67) are always a good start.

TENSION RELEASE

If you have a specific area of tension, you can help release it through breathing. Imagine that the energy of the breath is moving into the area of tension, with the tension flowing out on the exhalation. If it is muscular tension, and it feels okay to do so, deliberately tense that muscle group on the inhalation, holding briefly with tension, then let go of it on the exhalation (of course, using common sense: this may not be the best approach if the muscle is very sore or tender).

EARTHING BREATH

Another breath for letting go of stress and tension comes from the Taoist tradition. The idea of this is to let the stress or any negative emotions flow down through your body, through your legs and out through your feet into the earth. Taoists believe that the earth absorbs and recycles your negative energy like compost.

In this tradition, the point just below where the ball of your big toe meets the pad of the rest of the foot is called the 'bubbling spring' and it is thought that through this point the energy of the earth can bubble up into us and through it we can also let our stresses and negative feelings run down into the earth.

Sit comfortably with your feet flat on the floor and imagine on an in-breath that you are letting the energy of the earth flow up into you (the feeling is more like allowing it rather than forcing it). The energy flows up through the legs and into the body. On the exhalation let stress and tension flow out of your body, down through the legs and into the earth. Excess stress can flow down into the earth, just like an 'earth wire' conveys excess electricity.

THE PROJECTING BREATH

Another breath to release tension is to take a full breath and then purse your lips and strongly exhale. The opening is not tiny but small enough that the exhale takes a few seconds and feels as if this allows you to project your breath far from the body. The exhalation is strong (because the opening of the lips is restricted) but slow. The stress or tension can be sent out on the breath and can also be directed to trees — again, in the Taoist tradition there is the belief that trees take the stress and convert it into positive energy, just as they take carbon dioxide and convert it into oxygen.

Of course, you don't have to direct it towards trees; you can just breathe out. And if you aren't near any trees you can imagine one, or send it to a distant tree that you like and care about. These things work on many levels; even if the breath itself does not reach the distant tree, in the Taoist tradition there is a clear belief that some energy will reach it, and the practitioner will become more proficient in channelling and directing different energies. Also, if you picture sending the energy and feel the energy being sent it creates a psychological link to the distant tree, so you feel more connected to the living world around you. These links are good if you are feeling tense and a bit isolated, and you can also send it love. It is not in any way contradictory to send the negative energy along with love or gratitude, in the same way that you can care for a plant by fertilising it. I personally use this breath a lot if I feel any tension.

CIRCULAR BREATHING TO RELEASE EMOTION

One of the simplest ways to release emotion is to breathe in then release the breath out with no break in between. So the inhalation is controlled and the exhalation is passive. This is sometimes called 'circular breathing' (also described on p. 68). You only need a few breaths to feel you can release at least some of whatever emotion is concerning you, and you could overbreathe if you do it for too long — just pay attention to how you feel in doing it.

This type of breath has been often used in therapeutic 'breathwork', for releasing all sorts of emotional blockages.

The breath should be slow, not forced. If you practise this you are likely to find that the length of the passive exhalation varies a lot each time you do it — it is as if it acts to bring the emotions and the body back into balance.

This breath has the following aspects:

It is good to breathe in and out through the nose unless your nose is blocked. If your nose is blocked, breathe in and out through the mouth — having the breath go in and out through the same channel helps to balance it.

Don't breathe too much volume, just a comfortable, moderate amount. You will find it brings its own pace and balance, but start as slowly as feels comfortable.

9

ANXIETY, TRAUMA AND DEPRESSION

Breathing to overcome anxiety and panic

Breathing to overcome anxiety is essentially the same as breathing to calm (diaphragmatic breathing with extended exhalation, as on p. 66, or starting with belly breathing, on p. 64). Having worked with hundreds of people suffering anxiety conditions over the years, I can say that there are common breathing changes that happen to almost everyone when they are very anxious. Breathing becomes sharper and high in the chest, and either the person then holds the breath or their breathing rate escalates. These are distinct patterns without any depth of exhalation, and both keep the person stuck in the fight or flight anxiety state. I think this happens for almost everyone when they become anxious and it is certainly true for me. I notice if I feel stressed and anxious I often have a high breath and shallow exhalation.

To manage anxiety, it really helps to focus on the exhalation. If you can take a slow, deep, extended exhalation, you quickly begin to lower the anxiety level. 'Quickly' is a tricky word here, because when people are anxious they want to act quickly, to do rapid things to fix their anxiety and remove the threat. The rapid calm of breathing comes from breathing slowly and exhaling fully. It is rapid because in one or two breaths you can drop your anxiety level by 20 or 30 per cent. I say 20 or 30 per cent because in working with people suffering anxiety I often ask them to rate their anxiety on a scale of 1 to 10, where 1 is totally relaxed, like being at the beach on a warm summer's day, and 10 is totally overwhelmed by anxiety. It takes a few minutes to teach the technique but typically people will go from 7 to 5; 6 to 4; or occasionally 8 to 4. The amount of reduction averages about 30 per cent on the scale. Occasionally it takes someone a while to learn the breath, but once they are used to it, I find almost everyone can drop their anxiety rate by 2 points on the scale within a few breaths.

The key is to breathe diaphragmatically and slowly.

Jill

Jill saw me for social anxiety and performance anxiety. She was training in singing and of course knew diaphragmatic breathing well from her training. When I asked if she had ever used it to manage anxiety, she said no but was willing to try and could do it straight away without any coaching from me, other than to ask her to breathe slowly. She smiled and was surprised that it helped her feel much calmer. She went on to use it to good effect before social events, before performances and in breaks while performing.

If you are in an anxious state it is often easiest to learn belly breathing first (p. 64).

It helps to place one hand on your belly to help attend to the movement, and to squeeze in with the abdominal muscles to breathe out more fully, pushing in gently with the hand to aid the movement. The long exhale helps to activate the vagus nerve response so there is a physical sense of relaxing.

When you are anxious it is usually simplest to have the inhalation and exhalation the same length, but there is an option to extend the exhalation.

Breathing to stop panic attacks

Panic attacks can be terrifying — they are an extreme, powerful surge of anxiety. Typically in a panic attack, the person feels extreme anxiety and hyperventilates, breathing very fast and shallow. Often people fear that they are going to die, fearing heart attacks or complete collapse.

Using the breath is a powerful way to control and stop panic attacks. As a first step, it helps to recognize a panic attack for what it is. After you have one it is good to get a medical check to make sure that, for example, fear of having a heart attack is not because you are at risk of a heart attack. Once medical issues are ruled out, you can learn to recognize a panic attack when it happens and to know that it will pass. This acts to stop a common vicious cycle in which the initial anxiety kicks off a feeling of being anxious about being anxious, and panicking about the panic, so that everything worsens. Recognizing it means you can know it is unpleasant, but not ultimately harmful, and this helps it to pass more quickly.

One of the frightening things about panic attacks is that the hyperventilation produces very strong effects. Because you are breathing so fast, you breathe out way too much carbon dioxide, which results in less oxygen to the brain (as described on p. 34). This can lead to dizziness, trouble thinking clearly and a host of other symptoms.

In the middle of a panic attack slow, deep breathing will have a profound and positive effect, but generally you have to have a well-established breathing practice to be able to do it in the middle of a panic attack because the tendency to be caught in hyperventilation is very strong. It takes some muscular effort to control the breathing at a time like this. I can testify it works, but it is much better if you can you try to recognize the build-up to the panic attack. Then using slow, deep diaphragmatic breathing will be calming and prevent escalation. Once you do practice enough, however, you can control it even with an attack, but it takes enough practice to be able to take control of the muscles of breathing, which in this situation is challenging. One client, Penny, who had a history of panic attacks, found that she could develop control over her breathing, and found that it worked best for her to breathe in for a count of four then breathe out for a count of eight. She could stop the attacks within a minute.

Another option is to pause after the exhalation. This brings the carbon dioxide balance back up. This isn't always easy to do if you are panicking but it brings your system back into balance.

Breathing for post-traumatic stress

People who have suffered trauma often have a range of follow-on effects, from chronic tension to hypervigilance about any cues that remind them of the trauma, to bursts of rage or panic attacks. Some people I have seen for post-traumatic responses have a 'freezing up' of the diaphragm. In addition some trauma survivors unconsciously shut out body awareness — it is as if the body sensations themselves become associated with trauma. This can be true for survivors of childhood sexual abuse, victims of assaults or war veterans — the physical experiences were so horrific that there is a dissociation from feeling. Over time this can make the body itself feel like something 'other', something unknown and even hostile, responding at times unpredictably. While purposeful breathing can help, it needs to be a gentle and supportive process without pushing anything.

Some of the symptoms of PTSD can be helped with purposeful breathing for specific goals of calming or managing panic attacks as described elsewhere. If a post-traumatic memory comes up, the threat state can be reactivated in the here-and-now and long exhalations can help to move from fight or flight states to calm modes.

More broadly, though, it can be helpful to focus on having awareness in the body.

In recent years an approach has been developed called trauma-sensitive yoga.[1] In this very gentle approach the survivor is invited to make simple movements, usually while the facilitator is demonstrating the same movement. The focus is very simply on being aware of how it feels — having a safe context to begin to reconnect with embodied awareness, and slowly to become more and more comfortable with body awareness, in a real sense reconnecting with the body.

Slow, simple breathing with awareness can be part of this. It can be helpful to use any gentle controlled breath and just try to keep awareness in the body as you take the breath, noticing what moves, how it feels. The process is very much trying to stay with the sensations, in a gentle sensing mode of awareness as opposed to thinking about it, analyzing it or going off on other trains of thought.

This development of greater interoception and greater comfort from just being in the body has a healing effect.

Over time other steps can be taken, such as extending the range of the breath, breathing deeper and more diaphragmatically. Slowly, in safe steps, the body can be reclaimed, and hopefully, the simple joys of being in the body will become available again.

Josie

Josie had come in for help with post-traumatic stress.

Two years earlier she had had intruders break in to her home. There were several of them and it was a terrifying experience. Thankfully one of her family managed to phone the police and the intruders ran off without anyone having been assaulted. She had counselling afterwards, which was helpful for her. Recently she'd had a number of new stresses, including the death of a family friend and her grandmother becoming very ill. She had a recurrence of symptoms, said she could not stop worrying that something awful was going to happen, especially that her grandmother might die, and that she could not sleep. She was not getting more than two hours a night for days before coming in for help.

When asked where she was at this moment on a scale of 0 to 10, she said about an 8.5 or 9. I explained that slow diaphragmatic breathing was a helpful way to feel calmer and she was happy to try this in the session. After a few minutes of explaining it, demonstrating it and practising together I could see she looked more relaxed and asked where she was on the scale now, to which she replied a 5 or 6.

As Josie felt calmer, it was much easier to then look at other strategies as well, especially to review what was most helpful in her previous counselling, so as to access those resources again. She could begin to look in a more balanced way at acknowledging her present grief, anxiety and other worries, but with perspective and with options of how best to respond. She agreed to use the 'stop, breathe, refocus' strategy (see p. 90) with slow diaphragmatic breathing if she felt her anxiety rising, and also to use the same breathing style when lying down in bed at night.

Using the breath and building on cognitive skills from her previous therapy, Josie made rapid progress. At the third session two weeks later she said she had also been using the breath at night and sleeping much better, and if she felt anxious and stressed at night the breathing took stress from a 7 to a 3, after which she could usually drift off.

Maria

Maria saw me after having been in a car crash. She had post-traumatic symptoms including intrusive memories of the crash, nightmares, anxiety and avoidance of going in cars.

Among other things I talked with her about the links of breath with stress and emotions, and we practised the breathing with the intention of teaching her diaphragmatic breathing. This was initially was impossible for her; it was as if her diaphragm had completely frozen and her breath was high in the chest. Given this, we shifted focus to just breathing as slowly as she comfortably could and seeing if she could take the breath a little deeper as she practised. She found it difficult to take awareness into the body to notice just where the breath went, but could manage to slow her breathing down a little, and extend her exhalation a little in the session. I asked her to practise just doing a dozen breaths like this morning and night and whenever else she remembered and she agreed — just to try to gently extend the breath a little.

We had a session the next week and again the week after, and Maria was able to extend the breath and slowly begin to engage her diaphragm in the breathing — and as she did this she felt calmer. Over several sessions she extended this and we could do a systemic desensitisation in which she would just sit in a parked car doing this breathing to help calm herself, and then gradually building this step by step until she was able to both drive and be a passenger again.

Breathing for depression

Breathing styles linked with depression are more varied than those linked with anxiety because depression itself is generally more varied.

Depression is one word with many meanings, an umbrella term covering everything from 'feeling a bit flat', to 'a bad case of the blues', through to a complete immobilization requiring hospitalization. The extreme end of major clinical depression will require much more than simple breathing and has recently been found to have a range of very physical factors involved, often including inflammation of the brain.[2]

Breathing techniques can, however, be very beneficial in helping someone to be more energized, happier, 'get out of the slump' and also as part of a broader range of treatment for all levels of depression. The techniques can be a great way to lift yourself a little if you feel 'a bit depressed'. I also think it should be part of every assessment and treatment of depression. It is common in medical approaches to encourage people with severe depression to exercise, to socialize (not isolate themselves), to engage in positive activities and to ask about eating and sleeping patterns. All of these things are rightly seen as relevant factors and breathing should have no less a place in a plan of treatment.

Depression is usually multifactored and generally best seen as a bio-psycho-social condition. It is biological in that there are physiological changes in the body, particularly changes in brain chemistry. The most popular medications for depression boost the brain's serotonin, a neurotransmitter which is understood to be low in patients suffering depression. Exercise is also helpful in many ways, including affecting the balance of these brain chemicals, as it triggers a release of endorphins, which are linked with feelings of enjoyment.

Depression is also psychological in that the person's thoughts and feelings are very much affected. Cognitive behaviour therapy is the most widespread psychological treatment in recent times and this particularly addresses the person's thoughts, which tend to be distorted and unrealistically negative. Rumination, or thinking about negative things over and over, is a common factor in depression, and this can be changed. People's feelings are affected not only in the obvious sense of feeling bad, but also due to the tendency for different feelings to roll into one — so while the person might have reason to feel sadness, grief, resentment or other emotions, they tend not to be able to deal with them one by one but just feel an overall 'black cloud'. Counselling is often helpful to tease apart and acknowledge these feelings and enable them to be addressed. Each feeling on its own is much more manageable than all of them massed together.

Depression is social in that people often feel cut off from others and this may be exacerbated by relationship problems. It is also social in that the meanings we give to what is worthwhile, good or bad tend to derive from our culture and social groups, so the depressed sense of being a 'bad person' can link with comparing oneself to social norms and expectations.

Breathing can help the biological and psychological aspects and provide a way to interrupt negative thoughts, interrupt other patterns, raise energy and refocus.

Depression: a range of experiences and responses

One type of depression is being stuck with a deep sadness. In deep sadness there can be prolonged holding out of the breath.

Another is being anxious or stressed for so long that the system burns out. 'Burnout' is metaphorical, of course, but recent research supports this view. Another way to put it is that the system gets stuck on short circuit: fight or flight mode is switched on too long and the system becomes exhausted. There are some styles of breathing which are often helpful. One is deep, full breathing (p. 67), which helps to lift you a little, reducing the feelings of depression from, say, 7 to 5 on a scale of how you feel. Regular practice of slow, full breathing is likely to restore a sense of equilibrium and balance — the longer you continue the practice (over several days or weeks) the more effect it is gradually likely to have. Practising a restorative breath, especially the breaths per minute exercise on p. 73, is also likely to help. The more it is practised, the better.

Beyond these general guidelines, there can be some specific breaths that help to lift mood.

Interrupting depressed states

I have seen many people who have been depressed, very sad or grieving show a pattern of sighing deeply and holding the breath out. This reinforces a flattening of energy and a sense of stuckness. Changing the breathing pattern, such as using triangular breathing below, can help to lessen this.

TRIANGULAR BREATHING

Gently holding the breath can lift energy.

There should never be any strain, so the extent of the hold will vary. You should aim, however, to have the in-breath and out-breath the same length, and a hold in between. One ratio would be to breathe in for a count of four, hold the breath for up to a count of four (as long as it is comfortable), and breathe out for a count of four. If four is too long then in for four, hold for two and out for four; or in for six, hold for three and out for six. The number of the count does not matter — just keep a regular ratio. Do this for several rounds of breathing and finish the controlled breathing on an inhalation. Finishing the controlled breathing on an in-breath heightens energy a little — which is usually what you want with depression — while finishing on an out-breath flattens the energy a little.

It may sound a bit strange, but it is hard to feel quite so flat and down when you have taken a full breath and are holding it. When people are depressed they also tend to be stuck in depressive thoughts, and breath holding tends to lift people a little out of such thought loops.

Once you are lifted a little through the controlled breathing it becomes a bit easier to think about what is best to do. This may be to refocus on a task or to challenge depressing thoughts that are distorted. Sometimes this might be to recognize and acknowledge specific feelings that have fed into the general feeling of depression – some pain and sadness at times is part of life, but depression is often like a heavy blanket of feeling where all the bad feelings roll into one; separating these feelings out is helpful.

Radha

Radha had severe grief after the death of a very close friend. She had also suffered losses in her own family earlier in the year. She wept and clearly felt overwhelmed. We talked about her friend and the loss and about grief. During our session I told her at times to keep breathing. In the most intense feeling and weeping her breath would freeze. She would exhale in a deep sob and not inhale for some time, then gasp in the breath, sob out and not breathe in again for a time.

At a couple of points, I asked her to hold her breath. She did this and I asked her to hold it for as long as she comfortably could. This was surprisingly effective in lifting her out of the worst of the feeling. It seemed to clear her mind and allow her to refocus and talk things through more productively. I explained to her how, in grief and depression, people often hold the breath out, and how holding it in would help shift her out of the worst of it. I was careful to say that this was not a magic cure and would not stop the pain but would help her manage it better when she started to feel overwhelmed. This in turn helped us to move on to working together on grief counselling.

ARMPIT BREATHING

It is hard to be depressed if you are exposing your armpits.

If you feel down, sit or stand and extend your arms down by your sides, palms facing backwards. When you breathe in, raise your arms with the breath so that at the end of the breath your arms are up (and armpits exposed). As you exhale, slowly lower them again. Do several rounds. When I do this I find it hard not to smile. If I feel down it lifts me at least a little. It acts to open the front of the body and this has an uplifting effect.

One of the problems with being depressed is a lack of energy or motivation. So often people don't want to try something when they are flat. With this in mind, try the armpit breathing now, so you have at least tried it, and can use it as necessary at other times.

Justine

Justine came to see me for help with depression. She had been feeling flat and lethargic, finding it hard to get going. When I asked about breathing she said she had been taught a breathing technique, to breathe slowly as if into her belly. I said that was great that she had tried to do that and could pay attention to her breathing, but different styles of breathing were good for different effects, and while that one was best for managing anxiety, she might like to try a different one if she was feeling down.

We did both the full breath with a short retention and the armpit breath described above. I said to her that it is hard to be depressed when you are exposing your armpits and she was able to laugh a little. She liked the feeling of it and when I saw her again in a week's time, she said that she had used it during the week and found it helpful for lifting her mood and her energy.

PASSIVE SUPPORTED RESTING BREATH FOR DEPRESSION

If it feels too hard to do anything else, there are ways of resting which can help with depression.

When people are depressed they generally tend to slump forward, closing in their chest and reducing their breathing. A simple way to helpfully rest is to get a blanket (or two large towels) and fold it so that it forms a rectangle a couple of inches thick (you can play with the width and height to find the shape comfortable for you) and at least 1 metre (3 ft) long. Place it on the floor and lie on it, facing upwards with your spine along the blanket, with one end level with your lower back, just above the hips, allowing the natural curve of the spine, and with your head also on the blanket. You might also like a small pillow under your head. Let your arms rest on the floor out to your sides, at about a 30-degree angle, palms facing up. This gives a gentle passive opening to the chest. As you lie like this, do the full breath (p. 67) for several rounds and then relax, allowing your breathing to follow its own rhythm.

At the end, gently roll to your right-hand side, and rest a moment on your side before getting up.

Breathing can be linked with other interventions for depression, as in the case study below.

Carrie

Carrie, in her early twenties, was on antidepressant medication, which helped her manage her symptoms but did not stop her depression. She had issues related back to her childhood, particularly her parents' separation when she was eight. She felt abandoned by her father and missed him hugely. She saw him every second weekend but nonetheless had huge grief about his absence. Her relationship with her mother felt unsafe and her mother had drinking and drug problems and was involved with some people whom Carrie found threatening.

Carrie's recent problems had been sparked by insecurities after tension with her boyfriend and a falling out with her best friend.

She generally had good awareness of breathing, having played flute and done Pilates. Nonetheless this awareness did not carry over into the day-to-day. Her breath in the session was high, in the mid to upper chest, and had a 'gaspy' quality. She tended to have a long pause after exhaling. This type of breathing often happens with depression — it indicates a sense of feeling threatened, but also flat; anxious but worn out and de-energized.

Breathing, is, of course, only one aspect of the therapy, but in doing first diaphragmatic then full breathing Carrie felt more balanced, more energized and less down. With her background in other breathing techniques she learnt these instantly, and felt better when doing them. It was a practice she felt she would continue. In particular, Carrie recognized that if she felt 'flat' or felt that her 'insecurity issues' (as we agreed to call them) were triggered, she could name the feeling arising, take a few breaths, centre and stabilize, then refocus on what was best to do next. This also helped her to feel more confident in addressing the broader issues that challenged her.

10

ENHANCING ENERGY

To boost energy with breathing, you first have to pay attention to how you are breathing when you feel lacking in energy. For some people (maybe 10 per cent, but there are no definitive figures) this may be overbreathing, so they need to slow their breathing down. If you are already overbreathing, then pumping the breath to boost yourself will just throw your system more and more out of balance.

If you want to boost energy, first take a moment to check in with how you are breathing. If you are breathing through your mouth, chances are that you are overbreathing; by just switching to breathing through your nose for a couple of minutes you are likely to feel an immediate effect. If your nose is very blocked, then take a few breaths in which you purse the lips, breathing out slowly as if through a straw, slow the breath down and especially making the exhalation longer. This is likely to draw the system back to balance.

If you have been breathing through the mouth, breathing through the nose is likely to give a sense of clear headedness, as if the air itself was a type of subtle smelling salts. On the other hand, if your breathing has been more balanced and you want to pump up your energy, doing the *hara* breath (p. 104) in a muscular way for a few breaths tends to charge things up, with a quick hit of *prana*.

More generally, the full breath (p. 67) will bring a balanced sense of gently increasing energy. If you wanted more energy for working or doing a prolonged task, then the full breath would be ideal. Alternate nostril breathing (p. 80) for a few minutes is also a good option if you want a clear-headed subtly energized reset, such as for desk work.

THREE-PART BREATHING

Another good breath for energizing and building vitality is the three-part breath, known in yoga as *viloma*. In this breath the inhalation is interrupted and divided into three stages.

Do it gently, especially as you get used to it. First, breathe in to the lower section of the lungs (diaphragmatically) then pause for a second or so, then breathe to the middle, pause again, then complete the breath higher in the chest. Then breathe out gently, slowly and fully in one uninterrupted exhalation before breathing in the three-part breath again. Repeat for a few rounds. This has a gently energizing effect and in the longer term expands and extends breathing capacity.

A slightly more complex variation is to breathe in to the lower section for a count of three, pause for one count, breathe in to the centre for three, pause for one count, then breathe to the upper for three; then breathe out with a controlled exhalation to a count of nine. This generates extended breath control, but begin with the first variation.

Breathing to lift yourself up (or to stay awake)

Mostly the book has focused on helping people to be calmer, but breathing can also be used to subtly boost a sense of alertness. Some styles can give more of a quick hit of energy. Breathing to the upper chest tends to subtly stimulate the sympathetic nervous system, and this can be used to lift energy and stimulate yourself.

The full breath (p. 67) is one balanced way of doing this, but another is to deliberately breathe high and shallow to the upper chest. This type of breath for many people links with anxiety, but used with control it can also lift you up.

THE BIG SNIFF

Another subtle lift can come from a quick, strong snort through the nostrils. This takes the air over the front of the nostril area, which is subtly stimulating. I mentioned earlier that a great example of this was in the TV series, *The Borgias*, in which Jeremy Irons would sniff sharply and strongly when wanting to appear commanding. It conveyed an imperious quality of lifting above the throng, to clear the head and deliver a decisive edict.

In practice you can think of this as a big sniff, with the breath going to the upper chest, while lifting up and standing tall.

BREATH OF FIRE

While the big sniff gives a brief lift, to energize the whole system a great breath is the *hara* breath (p. 104). A strong related breath to pump you up is the 'breath of fire'.

Breathe in to the area just below and behind the navel, as described on p. 104. As you practise the breath, become more aware of the muscles involved, so you squeeze the air out by squeezing in the muscles of the belly and the navel area. The front of the belly moves a little, but does not just push out; the feeling is that the side and back muscles also move. On the inhalation the diaphragm moves down in the centre or back more than the front, and on the exhalation, squeeze in the muscles of the abdominal area.

As you practise the breath, become aware of making it more and more muscular, so the muscles become stronger and more practiced. The stronger and more muscular the breath the more energy it will generate. Make sure that as you breathe more quickly, the breath stays low and to the *hara* area (see p. 104). If you feel light-headed or a bit dizzy just stop and rest for a while, letting the breathing return to its own rhythm.

When done strongly and quickly, you will get a sense of the 'fire in the belly' charging up.

This breath only needs a few cycles — too much and you will overdo it. After a few rounds take a slower breath and allow a pause for a few seconds after the exhalation to restore the CO_2 levels a little.

A word on strong or gentle

A final word on breathing to boost energy. It is important to clarify that there is a big difference between a brief or time-limited burst of strong breathing and chronic overbreathing. It also requires a bit of self-awareness. If you overbreathe habitually, it will probably lead you to feel quite run down and then strong breathing won't help, as it is more of the same but cranked up; you would be better slowing the breathing down.

For a majority of people, though, if your energy is low then a few rounds of strong breathing can pump up the oxygen, help it flow through the body to where it is most needed and boost *ki/chi/prana*.

Breathing for clarity and focus

With any type of office work or study, it is important to take regular breaks, and purposeful breathing can be a means to feel more clear-headed. The type of breath you might best use will depend on how you feel at the time. If you feel tired and flat, an energizing breath will help. It is also good to get up and move around and some of the standing breaths (pp. 164–70) can be good options.

Taking the full breath (p. 67) is really good for being energized while calm and focused. Another great breath for office work or study is alternate nostril breathing (p. 80). This is traditionally used in yoga to bring the energies of the body into balance, and is claimed to bring the two hemispheres of the brain into balance. It produces a feeling of calm and balance, regardless of the underlying mechanism. Doing this breath for five minutes or more will bring a sense of clear-headedness and almost always a sense of being uplifted.

Alternate nostril breathing is especially helpful if you are feeling sluggish or finding it hard to focus.

Breathing to achieve goals

Simple breathing is a way to still the mind, so as to then focus on goals, especially as a prelude to visualization, which now has a large body of evidence to say that it can be a very powerful as a tool to work towards goals.[1]

A few rounds of slow, controlled breathing can help to settle the mind, and can help you enter a relaxed state that in many ways is similar to self-hypnosis. In these states the brain moves from the jumpy 'beta' brainwaves of everyday activity in to more 'alpha' brainwaves, linked with absorption, creativity and meditation.

Take a few full controlled breaths, to calm and centre, then let the breath become passive. In this state it can help to repeat a phrase that states your goal, or to visualize the goal, especially your ways of acting: picture what you will be doing once the goal is achieved, see yourself playing the game well, or speaking confidently or feeling relaxed or whatever is relevant for you.

While this sounds simple, it is very helpful. It is easy to think of a range of goals or have scattered thoughts, and simple visualization can help you focus. The brain in some ways doesn't know the difference between what you visualize and what you actually do, so the visualization is like an enacted practice.

Some of the best-selling self-help books in recent times have focused on the 'law of attraction', essentially saying that what you think about is what will manifest in your life.[2] This can be overstated, and much of the time people's thoughts are scattered and jumping around, so there could be a lot of random manifestations, but when you are deliberately calm and focused, setting an intention has a special power, reflected in changes in brainwaves. So use the breath first to calm you through slow, simple full breaths, then simply allow the breath to be passive and notice it, gently focusing awareness. This leads you into a very helpful meditative state of mind in which visualizing goals or repeating intentions has a special power.

Use simple intentions such as 'May I be peaceful and happy', 'May I be healthy', 'I shall … [adding your own goal]'. If you try to say this while you are sitting at the computer it will probably have little effect, but when sitting quietly and using the breath to calm and centre, it opens the way for this to have a real power.

Similarly, visualizing something you would like while in a calm state also has power — this might be performing well in sport, doing well in an exam, having confidence in giving a presentation. The method is very simple: just picture yourself doing whatever it is you want to do in the manner you want to do it. The link with breathing is that it is a bridge to the calm and centred state of mind needed for the directed imaging.

11

HEALTH AND PHYSICAL GOALS

Insomnia

There can be many causes of insomnia, but a common factor is difficulty 'switching off' before sleep. Many people who have difficulty getting to sleep report that their mind is still racing or churning over events that they are concerned about. When this happens it is often the case that the person is staying at least partly in a physiologically aroused (sympathetic nervous system) state, which is not compatible with sleeping.

Focusing on belly breathing (p. 64) or diaphragmatic breathing (p. 65) can help with this. I have worked with many people who have found it makes a big difference just to lie in bed on their backs, with one hand on their belly. In this breath, just focus on *breathing in, the hand goes up; breathing out, the hand goes down.* Just focusing on the breath tends to act to slow the breathing down, but you can consciously also slow the breath down, just as much as is comfortable, or to five or six breaths per minute.

Doing belly breathing switches on the rest and relax (parasympathetic) response of the body, which helps you relax ready for sleep. It also gives the mind a focus, so rather than thinking about worries it switches out of 'talking and thinking mode' into 'sensing and body awareness mode', and this aids the shift into letting go for sleep. Further to this, it helps to know that even if you don't get quickly to sleep, being in this type of mode allows the body to be relaxed and to gain many of the benefits of sleep — the rest mode allows body repair and the meditative quality of simple breath awareness has many healing benefits. Recognizing this helps in that it also takes the struggle out of getting to sleep. Most people are aware of the paradox that you cannot force yourself to go to sleep, and the more you try the harder it gets. Going to sleep is a process that happens by allowing it, and letting go. That is why some old fashioned distraction techniques can be helpful, like counting sheep. Focusing on very simple belly breathing, feeling comfortable that the process itself is helpful for rest and repair, also allows the mind to let go.

While slow, deep, diaphragmatic breathing is usually best for sleep, a friend of mine recently reminded me of how important it is to pay attention to your own styles and what works for you. He is very successful and very hard-working and switching off from the many demands upon him can be an issue. He found that at night alternate nostril breathing really helped him to get off to sleep. This is a bit unusual as many people find it calming but mildly stimulating. My sense is that for him it allowed a letting go of the left-brain problem-solving function for a while, bringing the hemispheres into balance. The greater complexity of this breathing style may also have helped him to keep more focus upon it, rather than drifting back to thinking of work decisions. Whatever the reason, it works, and is a good example of how to adapt what works for you with some small experiments and attention to your own responses.

Breathing for better health

The first step in breathing for better health is to check first whether you have any problem styles of breathing and to correct these.

Reverse breathing and constricted breathing are both common and engaging the diaphragm will make a big difference. Overbreathing is also common and often linked with breathing through the mouth. If you breathe through the mouth, shifting to nostril breathing will make an immediate difference. If you find it hard to breathe through the nostrils, such as due to congestion, then be gentle with it, and just move over time to more nostril breathing. As you stay with it, the nostril breathing itself is likely to have the effect of reducing the congestion. If you have been breathing through the mouth, gently reducing the amount of breath may be helpful.

One of the best breaths for general health, though, is a slow deep inhale, making sure to use the diaphragm and then letting the air gently fill the chest and then a slow passive exhalation. Focus on trying to breathe in and out for five or six seconds (so at five or six breaths per minute, as feels best for you — or as slowly as feels comfortable if that feels too slow for you). This slow, deep breathing has an effect of bringing everything into balance.

Less is often more

Better health won't be achieved by a few breaths. While most of the focus of this book is on immediate change, using specific breaths to rapidly achieve a change of mood or mode, better health is linked to a change in your day-to-day breathing pattern. This can be profound but is a slower process to longstanding change by implementing a few core ideas and practices.

The volume of air we breathe is a very important factor, as discussed in Chapter 2, and one that can vary hugely depending on our activity level. The amount of air going in and out is referred to as the tidal volume, and this is multiplied by the number of breaths per minute to calculate the minute volume (volume of air going in and out each minute). The average rate of breathing varies but is typically about twelve breaths per minute at rest. So with an average of 0.5 litres per breath, the minute volume at twelve breaths per minute, would be about 6 litres. This is about what most medical textbooks would say is normal and healthy.

In a review of the scientific literature, Dr Artour Rakhimov compiled figures for rates of breathing. Research participants with health conditions (people with heart disease, diabetes, sleep apnoea and asthma) all had minute volumes over 14, while people with cancer and panic disorder had minute volumes over 12.[1] While of course some conditions may cause problematic breathing rather than be caused by it, there are remarkable links between overbreathing and many medical conditions.

Some of the original research leading to awareness of less being more was conducted by Russian Professor Konstantin Buteyko. During his medical studies he was assigned the task of monitoring the breathing patterns of patients with different conditions at a medical institute in Moscow. He particularly spent time sitting with dying patients and recorded clear patterns related to breathing and different conditions, especially noting acceleration of breathing prior to death. Somewhat macabrely, he could predict how long it would be before someone would die by noting how excessive their breathing had become.

Buteyko theorized that the excessive breathing led to lower CO_2 and in turn less release of oxygen through the body, and that this might lead to a range of difficulties and diseases. He himself suffered from hypertension, and decided to measure his own CO_2 levels and modulate them through controlled breathing exercises, especially reducing the amount of breathing. He effectively cured his own condition and then conducted experiments related to a range of other conditions. His breathing techniques are best known for helping asthma. The main focus of the approach is to help people reset their basic rate of breathing, with the central focus on reducing overbreathing.

Whether overbreathing or underbreathing, the more you can be aware of the breath the better, in particular being aware that breathing at rest does not require a lot of air exchange. A small tidal volume at twelve breaths per minute is fine.

You can gently tune in to this by breathing through the nose, to allow a natural breath — not breathing in forcefully, just feeling as if you allow the breath, and allowing a pause after the exhalation, and generally, having the breath be soft, gentle and easy. You can follow the instructions for the simple meditative breath on p. 73. As you do this you will probably find the breath slows down to find its own balance.

For long-term health and to immediately feel good, engage the diaphragm and take full breaths for about five or six breaths per minute. If this is too slow for you, then just slow down as much as is comfortable. This brings the system into balance and is especially good for consciously breathing for a few minutes any time you have a break in the day, for an immediate sense of calm and poise.

Longer term, slow, gentle, relaxed breathing is good for everyday life. This can be practised by nose breathing, with gentle inhalations engaging the diaphragm, passive exhalation and natural pauses in the breath. In the sixth century BC, Chinese philosopher Lao Tzu summed this up by saying, 'The perfect man breathes as if he is not breathing'.

Breathing for healing

As well as a general breath for better health, breathing can aid healing in several ways.

- Simple slow, deep diaphragmatic breathing (p. 65) will help as it puts the body into rest and repair (parasympathetic) mode.
- Breathing at about the six breaths per minute rate seems also to help bring the body into balance, enhancing healthy heart responses.
- Using the breath as a way to find deep relaxation will aid the healing process.
- If a particular part of the body needs healing, breathe in while imagining the energy of the breath moving to that part. Eastern approaches have long accepted that this sends life energy to the area. Western understandings are less clear, but this practice can increase blood flow to the

area, and is likely to help reduce inflammation. You can imagine the breath's energy, on the inhalation, going to the affected area as a white light; then on the exhalation any stress or negativity can be imagined to be breathed out like a grey mist.

Slow, deep, gentle and still a little mysterious

Slow, deep and gentle breathing has a range of health benefits, from balancing sympathetic and parasympathetic activity to heart health, stress reduction and all the benefits that go with less stress. Other health benefits are still being identified. Recent research has found that yoga breathing stimulates nerve growth factor, which is important in the growth, development and maintenance of a healthy nervous system.[2]

More broadly, a recent scientific review entitled 'The physiological effects of slow breathing in the healthy human' states that 'the physiological effects of slow breathing are indeed vast and complex' and several reviews show that the physiological mechanisms are remarkably still being mapped out.[3,4]

Breathing for pain management

Pain has a helpful purpose: to alert us to problems. So the first thing with pain management is always to make sure the pain is not signalling that something needs medical attention.

Having said that, breathing to manage pain has long been used in Eastern traditions.

Pain has several components:

- whatever is happening at the site of the pain, including strain or inflammation and the responses of the nerves there
- the processing of the signals from the local nerves in the

brain itself; for chronic pain, often an oversensitivity develops in the relevant area of the brain
- the emotional reaction, which is the sense of suffering
beyond the simple physical sensations
- the thoughts associated with the pain
- any compensatory adjustments, such as tensing muscles to
protect the painful area.

While purposeful breathing can't cure the core physical problem, it can help with this cluster of interrelated responses.

One of the best techniques is to imagine the energy of the breath going to the area that is painful, and then imagine any of the pain and tension flowing out on the out-breath.

A second way to help chronic pain is to be aware that pain always involves the site of the pain but also the brain's processing of the signals of pain. Using slow, deep diaphragmatic breathing (p. 65) to switch out of fight or flight and into a relaxed state will help the whole nervous system response to calm. This should help the pain feel more manageable.

Mindfulness meditation (pp. 150–52) has been very well used in recent years as an aid to managing chronic pain.[5] Practising just noticing the breath is a form of this meditation and can be carried over to noticing the pain as just a physical sensation. This pure sensation is often made much worse by the sense of emotional suffering that often accompanies it, so just noticing the sensation has a positive effect, making it more manageable.

Best breathing during exercise

Having begun the introduction to this book with my question to my football coach, it is worth mentioning that I have found ways of breathing that are better for exercise and which I find give more endurance.

The basic mechanics of breathing make a big difference. If you are breathing high in the chest, it is going to dramatically cut down fitness. When people only breathe to the upper chest, they only use a fraction of their capacity, and are using supporting muscles to achieve the breath and these can quickly tire. If they are 'reverse breathing' (p. 51) it will both cut down fitness and throw out coordination.

As long as the breathing is primarily diaphragmatic, it is going to help exercise. If the main muscle group designed for breathing (the diaphragm) is being used it prevents overtaxing secondary muscles, and more energy is then available for the rest of the body.

In strong exercise a good option to build on this is the *hara* breath (p. 104). Breathing strongly to the hara tends to build energy. The *hara* breath implicitly engages more the back of the diaphragm area, which feels efficient and centring.

For the most part, you do not need to focus on pumping more air though the body. If you are exercising hard you need to be sensitive to the needs of your body, but slow, steady, deep breathing is usually enough. In yoga, even in quite strenuous movement routines the emphasis is on the breath being slow and controlled.

Really pumping the breath is only required at extremes. For this, there can be training to use all the muscles involved in breathing as a 'breathing pump'. This training can include strengthening these muscles by breathing against resistance (using a device designed to make it harder to breathe so the muscles have to work more).[6] This training will make a difference in the last 200 metres of your Olympic rowing final, but is less relevant to the weekend athlete. Having said that, if you are in a cycling group on Sundays, a strong related breath can be a two-part inhalation — strongly to the *hara* and then to the chest, and then a two-part exhalation from chest and belly. It is a simplified 'pump' in which you can feel the pumping action.

Breathing to cool down

If you are feeling overheated on a hot day or after exercise, a helpful breath to cool down is to open your mouth and curl your tongue (so it forms a 'U' in the 'O' of your mouth). Breathing in so the air flows over your tongue has a very cooling effect. It is one of very few yoga breaths in which you breath in through the mouth.

If you have trouble curling your tongue, don't worry: there is a genetic capacity (or lack thereof) to be able to do this curling. For those folks who are genetically challenged in the tongue-curling department (like me), breathing over the tongue with the air coming through a small pursed-lip opening of the mouth has much the same effect. You can feel the air being cool on the surface of the tongue as you breathe in.

Another cooling option from the yoga traditions is to have the teeth touching and then breathe through the teeth. This is the recommended yoga form for those who can't curl their tongue, but I prefer just breathing over the tongue through the narrow mouth opening.

Breathing to lose weight

Okay, the old saying really is true that 'Man cannot live by breath alone' (or was that bread?).

While there are reports of mystics in the Himalayas living on the energy of the breath alone, the rest of us mere mortals need a healthy diet.

Where purposeful breathing can be helpful with weight loss is firstly as an alternative to snacking. If you feel like a snack, why not spend a couple of minutes doing your favourite breathing technique instead? If you are really ravenous, this won't be foolproof but a lot of calories are taken in from snacks we don't really need. Stopping and doing some deep breathing interrupts the urge and feels good. A particular breath can be to breathe deeply down the back of the body, then forcefully exhale from the belly, squeezing in the abdominal muscles. This has a good effect of interrupting any urges to snack. It allows you to 'stop, breathe, refocus' away from food.

Managing appetite can also be influenced by calm, slow steady breathing in which CO_2 levels are not depleted. If you are overbreathing you are more likely to feel agitated and also hungry. Slow, gentle breathing with long exhalations and pausing with the breath out allows a slight build-up of CO_2, while still having ample oxygen. This has a calming effect and the CO_2 relaxes the smooth muscles of the gut, which helps you feel less hungry.

I find it really effective if I can sit quietly and breathe in strongly for a count of four, gently out for a count of eight and then pause for a count of four with the breath out. This is very calming and has the effect of stilling any hunger. This count may be a bit too slow for a beginner, and needs to be done without any strain, so it feels very comfortable, but you can adjust the count to suit yourself, while keeping the general ratio of shorter inhalation, longer exhalation and a retention of the exhalation, holding the breath out for a short pause.

Beyond specific breaths, a lot of excessive eating can be emotionally driven, when feeling bored or down in some way. Stopping and doing a few minutes of breathing and simple meditation (such as on the breath or mantra) allows a sense of connecting with yourself in a positive and peaceful way.

Another important point is that a lot of eating for most people is done mindlessly, and eating mindfully is being shown in many psychology studies to make a real difference. Basically, this is really paying attention to what you eat when you are eating (as opposed to eating while watching TV or doing another task, or thinking of other things). If you give your full attention to what you are eating, you are likely to both enjoy the food more and be satisfied with a smaller portion. A student of mine recently said she had been practising mindful eating and by just doing this for a couple of weeks had lost several kilos. Breathing can play a role just by taking a couple of slow, controlled breaths before you eat in order to help calm and focus.

Of course, healthy eating is always central. Like exercise, breathing skills can be part of a weight loss program, but should not be used obsessively. It can be an aid to a balanced diet, not a replacement.

12

HAPPINESS, INSPIRATION, CREATIVITY

Often, feeling happier can be simply linked to getting out of stress states. Once we have switched on the calm response with slow, deep breathing the body moves to a more relaxed and contented state.

It does seem that we are 'hardwired' for happiness, as long as we are removed from threat. Being removed from threat is not as simple as it sounds, because the sense of threat may be carried in our thoughts, and stresses can come from so many sources in the modern world. Any of the styles of breathing with meditative awareness (see Chapter 13) can allow a tuning in to a deeper sense of calm, as can the breathing style below.

INNER SMILE BREATHING

A beautiful style of breathing for enhancing happiness comes from Esoteric Taoism.

Sit comfortably on a chair, keeping your back straight. Close your eyes and gently smile. Try to feel the smile in your eyes and let the corners of the mouth gently pull upwards. Mostly this is subtle and the movement is quite small. This gentle smile sets off a cascade of neurochemicals that link with feeling happy and peaceful. It is a form of sending love to yourself. If you try too hard to move the muscles of the mouth and eyes you can lose this, so play with it a little. This is also a beautiful way to let go of stress and negativity. Once you have the feeling of the smile, allow it to spread down through your body, moving through each organ or area with the in-breath and then spreading through that area on the out-breath (or alternatively, letting any tension flow out on the exhalation).

Another option to generate the same effect is to close your eyes and imagine someone or something you love in front of you (this might be your romantic partner, your child or parent, a religious figure or a scene from nature). Let yourself smile at him/her/it. Really try to feel the smile and imagine projecting loving energy. Then let that loving energy move from your eyes to spread down through your face, then neck, then body. With each in-breath feel and imagine the energy building, and with each out-breath let the loving energy spread to your body bit by bit.

A variation is to take this energy through the whole body on the in-breath and imagine every cell being filled, vibrating with the loving energy on the out-breath, as if every cell is dancing with energy.

The old saying that it takes many more muscles to frown than to smile, has truth in it. Beyond that, however, smiling sets off a flow of healing energy, and emotional and neurochemical changes in ways that are very simple but quite beautiful.

Breathing and inspiration

It is no coincidence that the word 'inspiration' means both to literally breathe in and also to be filled a higher insight, energy or purpose. The

Oxford English Dictionary defines inspiration as 'a breathing in or infusion of some idea, purpose, awakening, or creation of some feeling or impulse, especially of an exalted kind'.

Throughout history, 'inspiration' in its broader sense has two further distinct but overlapping meanings in both the arts and spiritual realms. The first is the creative moment. The other meaning is the broader one of being infused with a new sense of purpose, meaning or direction — to be uplifted and reinvigorated, to have our spirits filled anew. This almost always entails connecting with something bigger than our usual sense of self, so that there is a sense of expansion and connection with something greater, whether in a spiritual sense or connection with an ideal or environment.

The two meanings can overlap, such as when a new insight is linked with a sense of happiness, joy and vitality. After all, if we have a creative thought but can't be bothered acting on it, it is not inspiration. Nonetheless the focuses are different, so are explored separately here.

Breathing and the creative moment

In ancient times, inspiration was always seen to come from outside the individual, from the gods or muses. The ancient Greeks saw that a poet would be seized by a divine madness — the *furor poeticus* — as inspiration flowed through them. Roberto Calasso, in his book on ancient Greek mythology, *The Marriage of Cadmus and Harmony*, says that the ancient Greeks had no interest in anything similar to modern psychology. Calasso says that the Greeks saw individuals as mundane, and that people only did exceptional things when under the influence of the gods, therefore it was only the gods that were worth studying. Inspiration came from outside and infused us.

From a modern Western perspective, inspiration more often comes from within, and one of the major studies of creativity done in recent years was by Mihaly Csikszentmihalyi, published in his book *Creativity: Flow and the psychology of discovery and invention*.

The study looked at the creative breakthroughs of famous scientists, artists and businesspeople. What Csikszentmihalyi calls the 'aha' experience almost always seemed to come at a moment when the person concerned had taken time away from their work and was relaxed. He suggested that 'the insight presumably occurs when a subconscious connection between ideas fits so well that it is forced to pop out into awareness, like a cork held underwater breaking out into the air after it is released'.[1] It is said to follow an 'incubation' time, typically one in which after working intensively on a project a person then rests, relaxes, 'switches off' the conscious focus of work or has some 'idle time'. In this way the 'backdrop' of thinking, the immersion in the field, the dedication to the problem and the motivation to achieve a breakthrough are all important background factors, but the moment of inspiration is found in stillness or when idly focused elsewhere.

The concept of 'modes' is relevant here. When people feel threatened there is generally a narrowing of attention, so relaxed modes are important for inspiration. Secondly, inspiration often arises in changing modes. If you are working hard for too long, eventually you begin to feel exhausted and robotic, and it is unlikely much inspiration will arise. Having a break and some time in stillness, or just allowing thoughts to flow idly is likely to allow new connections and creative insights to emerge. On the other hand, if you spend all you time idling, you are likely to get lazy and inspiration will be even less likely to arise. It is in moving between these states that creative insight is likely to occur.

SETTING AN INTENTION

A helpful way to invite inspiration can be to set an intention, focus clearly upon it, and then let it go and be still and 'empty'. Being empty is surprisingly difficult so a more focused way, using the breath, is to do the following.

Set an intention, focus clearly upon it, and then let it go. Do a few rounds of controlled breathing and then let the mind be still or quietly absorbed in simple awareness, such as awareness of the breath. Notice any thoughts, words or images that arise. Let the mind be empty as much as you can but if the mind wanders (which it is bound to from time to time) gently draw it back to the breath.

Inspiration can never be forced, but this seems a powerful way to invite it. It is surprising how often something helpful 'bubbles up' to help resolve a work problem or life dilemma, or to help you find a renewed sense of direction.

Breathing and feeling inspired

Historically, feeling inspired has been seen in religious terms of being inspired by God or the gods, wanting to emulate the saints or be filled with divine spirit. These meanings are still present but in the modern, secular world the idea usually has a broader meaning of being inspired by an ideal, a higher purpose or by a role model. It is a connecting with an idea, ideal or purpose which is uplifting, a joyful motivation and sense of transcending the mundane. Almost always it is linked with connecting with something bigger, whether spiritually or some other greater good, rising above the ordinary.

Where the breath can link with this is in centring and refocusing. Most of us will have some experience of having felt inspired or uplifted and having higher goals with which we can identify, but often it is hard to maintain focus on these things amidst the stresses and myriad demands of everyday life. Many people find there is so much clutter that higher purposes become lost.

BREATHING INTO INSPIRATION

Taking some full breaths to centre, allow the breath to become passive; this can allow a stillness of mind and then a focus can be given to reconnecting with higher goals and values (see also p. 90). Remind yourself of these goals and values, such as to love and be loved, to help others, to find truth and beauty, to reach your full potential. This can be energizing at a deep level, aligning with inspiring goals.

Taking in energy

Another practice is to imagine a source of inspiration as divine energy. In most spiritual traditions there is ultimately a source of highest energy and highest consciousness; of infinite energy and consciousness, with the energy being both uplifting and loving. Different traditions might call on this through the many names of the divine. Christians might think of the Holy Spirit permeating creation. Others might think of the Universal Energy, Great Spirit, Brahman or more metaphorically as sunshine or a white light.

ENERGY AS INSPIRATION

A meditative breathing practice is to imagine divine energy being drawn into the body with every in-breath — not just through the nose or mouth but through every pore of the body, infusing every cell. On the out-breath, allow every cell to be filled, as if smiling and vibrating with the energy, then filling again with the in-breath.

At the end of the practice, make sure to allow yourself a few minutes to just sit quietly, letting the breath be passive. Finish with a gentle thought of thanks to this highest energy and consciousness, however you have conceptualized it.

Breathing for flow states

When people are performing at their best, whatever their field of endeavour, they often describe being 'in the zone' — a state of being fully absorbed and focused. Psychologist Mihaly Csikszentmihalyi describes these as 'flow' states, in which someone fully applies themself and is fully engaged in the task.[2] In this state there is a loss of any self-consciousness and the state is very satisfying. Whether an athlete performing at her peak, an artist painting, a chef creating gourmet food or someone fully engrossed in their day-to-day work, this is a state of productivity, which is enjoyable for its own sake.

Typically, this state involves tasks in which the level of challenge is not too low (leading to boredom) or too high (perhaps leading to frustration or anxiety). You would not be focused on your breathing, as it would distract you, but breathing can be a helpful tool for helping to prepare for tasks in which you would like to be 'in the zone'. A few controlled breaths before engaging in the task can help to still the mind, centre the focus, first on the breath itself but then, when the mind is focused, on the task you are about to engage in. You can also be aware of where you want to be on the scale (like the Yerkes-Dodson scale on p. 100) of physiological activation — too low and you won't perform well; too high and you may have trouble focusing. Remember as well that some stress can be a good thing if you can direct your focus and use it (channeling it like an athlete). Once you are used to recognizing your own states of activation, then you can use the different breaths described in the book to pump yourself up a little more or calm yourself down to be ready to focus with best efficacy.

PART 4

Meditation, mindfulness and Eastern traditions

13

BREATHING AS A MEANS OF MEDITATION

Meditation can sometimes sound mysterious but in its essence is a very simple practice. Simply focusing on the breath is itself a form of meditation.

Meditation's forms may vary but they all have common themes. A comparison can be made with exercise. Exercise can vary from going for a walk, to running a race, playing tennis or pumping iron at the gym. The commonality is physical exertion of one form or another. Meditation has the common feature of stilling the mind to give attention to one simple focus. This can be simple awareness of the breath, focus on a sound or image, body awareness or an open stillness — letting the mind be empty and noticing whatever thoughts or sensations come into awareness. Part of meditation is a process of noticing when the mind wanders and gently drawing attention back to the initial focus.

While an ancient practice, meditation has become very popular in the West in recent years and well accepted in Western medicine. Programs such as Jon Kabat-Zinn's mindfulness-based stress reduction are now offered in hospitals and clinics around the Western world, and mindfulness techniques have become a central feature of many schools of modern psychology.

Mindfulness

Mindfulness is a skill that is usually taught as a form of meditation and can easily follow on from controlled breathing.

Mindfulness is a form of 'bare attention' in which awareness is directed to the person's present experience. In the practice described below, the awareness is directed to the breath, or more broadly to the body (as opposed to, say, being 'lost in your thoughts' about what's happening on the weekend or thinking about work). The aim is to simply notice, giving your full attention to your present experience. One technique sometimes used in teaching mindfulness is to have you simply eat a single raisin, taking three or four minutes to do so (as opposed to quickly chomping a handful). The exercise has you initially just hold the raisin in your mouth, feeling its texture, noticing any responses such as saliva being released, then slowly biting it, noticing textures and tastes, gently chewing it or rolling it around the mouth and so on until it is swallowed. The idea is that when full awareness is given to this, something so simple takes on a very different dimension.

In Buddhist practice mindfulness is often practised by quietly noticing whatever comes into your awareness. Often the meditator might name the thoughts or sensations as they arise. This form of mindfulness can be done when sitting, walking around or in doing simple tasks. This practice of simply noticing the thoughts and sensations allows you to notice reactions, feelings and thoughts which are otherwise often 'just below the surface'. Such noticing without responding can have a remarkably freeing effect. Buddhist psychology holds that this type of attention in itself is healing.

The practice of mindfulness allows you to become more aware of your thoughts and to then separate yourself from these thoughts. We all have patterns of responding to different events and some of these patterns are outside of conscious awareness. This awareness gives you more choice in how to respond to different situations. For someone who is depressed or anxious, noticing the thoughts and various embodied responses allows a recognition that the thought is 'just a thought', rather than something compelling.

MINDFUL AWARENESS OF THE BREATH

One of the most popular forms of mindfulness is to take the awareness to the breath and/or body. You might like to read then practise the format described here.

Close your eyes and be aware as you do this that closing the eyes is a sign of taking the awareness inwards. Allow your awareness to go to your breath. Simply notice your breath. There is no need to control or direct it. Notice it however you notice it, whether this is the rise and fall of your chest, movement of your belly or subtle movement of your back, the passage of air through your nose or throat. If any thoughts come into mind, just notice them and let them pass and draw your attention back to your breath. After a while let your awareness go through your whole body. Notice any body sensations. Simply notice them, there is no need to change anything, just simply be aware. Stay with this for a few minutes.

An important part of the practice is to be aware that thoughts are likely to come and go, even for the most experienced meditator. When you become aware that you have wandered off on a train of thought, simply notice the thought and let go of it, and gently draw your awareness back to the breath. This noticing and letting go of thoughts is an important part of the process.

Mindfulness tends to have the dual benefits of being calming and also, over time, helps develop a greater capacity to become aware of cognitions, emotions and modes of being in everyday life. This is helpful for many things, including managing stress and directing your attention in the best way for different situations. Particularly when people are anxious, stressed or depressed they tend to have a lot of thoughts that are anxious, stressful or depressing. Having a mindful awareness of these helps to make the thought just a thought and to let it pass or be there in the background; you can then refocus and get on with whatever it is you want to do. Noticing breathing patterns can also be part of this awareness and then the option is available to use purposeful breathing to reset.

Benefits of mindfulness

The last couple of decades have seen an explosion of research into the benefits of mindfulness, and it has become very much a part of mainstream psychology practice.

These benefits include reducing stress, improving wellbeing, increasing emotional regulation, better management of pain, helping in the treatment of depression, facilitating post-traumatic growth, building self-compassion, improving general health, improving academic performance, improving work performance and increasing resilience. It has also been shown to produce a raft of very positive changes in the brain, increasing both the size and functionality of areas of the brain associated with cognition, emotional regulation, learning and memory.[1]

Breathing and mantra for relaxation

Mantra is a form of meditation which involves the repetition of sound. While this has a long tradition in the East, one of the most influential Western researchers, who has since the 1970s promoted the importance of deep relaxation, is Herbert Benson, whose original book was entitled *The Relaxation Response.*[2]

Benson teaches a way of relaxing that involves sitting comfortably, relaxing as much as possible from the feet through the whole body to the head, then breathing slowly and silently repeating a simple word or sound in your mind. For Benson it was clear that the specific word or sound did not really matter — it could be 'one', 'peace', 'love', 'calm' or anything that had a positive or neutral connotation. For Benson, the word or sound was silently repeated but you can also say it aloud. When thoughts come up, as they inevitably will from time to time, just notice them, let them pass and return to the repetition of the word or sound. This is a very simple way to calm and deeply relax, which has been also very well researched.

Breathing with sound

In yoga traditions mantra has a special place. The physical *asana* (poses and postures) and breathing practices of yoga help prepare for meditation. Many yoga classes that focus on *asana* will also include some *pranayama* (controlled breathing) and meditation at the end of the class.

Mantra meditation has been practised in India for millennia, and specific mantras are often assigned by a spiritual teacher to a disciple. The most central and widely used mantra in the yoga traditions is *om*, which is now very widely known in the West as well as the East. *Om* sits within a spiritual tradition and is seen to signify the divine, and the universal vibration or energy which underlies all creation. Repeating the mantra is traditionally seen as bringing us more in tune with this energy. *Om* repetition has also been scientifically researched in recent years as a practice for general well-being, with many benefits and being safe to practice, though these studies are mostly within a cultural context which respects its spiritual aspects.[3] It is best learnt and practised within a broader spiritual framework.

A related practice is just to hum the 'mmm' sound. In yoga there is a practice called *brahmari mudra*, in which the ears are gently blocked by pushing in on the small protruding piece of cartilage at the front of the ears (the tragus) while humming the 'mmm' sound, said to be like the buzzing of bees. This gentle pushing on the tragus to block the ears magnifies the effect of the humming. The practice is linked with a wide range of helpful applications, from relaxation to ease of childbirth. It is considered safe, except that it might be best avoided if you have tinnitus.

'MMM'

Simple humming of the 'mmm' sound without blocking the ears is also a good practice. Another great alternative is to repeat 'hum' so that the 'hu' is relatively brief and most of the practice is the 'mmm' sound. This simple humming, with a long 'mmm' on a slow gentle exhalation, has physical effects and effectively provides a subtle 'brain massage', as the brain gently vibrates with the sound. You can feel this subtle vibration as you practise. Some of the vibration directs to the pituitary gland (which sits roughly above the top of the back of the mouth, above the soft palate). This gland is the 'master gland' which affects the balance of release of all the hormones, so the gentle vibration acts as a tonic for the whole system. Different traditions have different emphases of pronunciation and different intonations can gently direct the vibration to different areas of the brain.

Simply sit quietly with the spine straight and slowly, gently, softly recite 'hum' or 'mmm'. This humming type of sound makes intuitive sense to anyone who has hummed a happy song. Like slow breathing itself, repeating slow, gentle humming on a long exhalation is something easily available but which most people would never think to do. A few simple breaths like this can feel quite uplifting and profoundly peaceful. There is a sense for most people of feeling more centred afterwards and more generally 'in tune'.

SO-HUM

Another calming, centring meditation is to gently in your mind say the sound 'so' on the inhalation, with no external sound beyond the sound of the breath itself, and 'hum' on the exhalation. This is traditional and very peaceful.

The meaning of the words is 'I am That', an identification with the divine, from traditions that believe all of us have a spark of the divine within us. Regardless of your personal beliefs there is a meditative effect from the practice.

The mantra of great happiness

There are many different mantras for many different purposes, but one of my favourites is the mantra of great happiness. This is *Om maha aham*. *Om* is the universal vibration linked with many mantras, *maha* means great and *aham* here connotes happiness, or more strictly 'I am' or 'I am That', like so-hum.

When chanting *om maha aham* I always want to smile, partly because 'aha' and *aham* seem to have a universal sense of surprise and realization. The 'a' sounds are soft — like 'ah', closer to the sound in 'hum', not like the 'a' in 'jam'. Like all mantras it works on the quality of the vibration that the sounds produce, rather than any literal meaning of the word — it is a felt experience, not an intellectual one.

Meditation and the pleasure dial

One of the benefits of meditation is that it brings a sense of very pleasurable peace and calmness. This is not to say that every mediation session will produce this — some may have some sense of restlessness or discomfort, or perhaps unresolved feelings may arise. But generally, as people meditate more the sense of peace and calm feels good. There is a sense that underneath all the clutter and clamour of everyday life there is a deep wellspring of peace, that can flow through each of us if we are just still enough to allow it.

There can be different ways to understand this. For some it will be that we are more in tune with the loving energy of a universal spirit, but for others it can just be that our systems are basically geared to be gently, peacefully happy if we have time enough away from stress or threat.

Meditation allows a sense of decluttering the mind so we become more in tune with deeper or higher aspects of ourselves. Many people have told me that for them life just flows better when they meditate — they are more intuitive and more able to respond to what is important, clearer-headed and feel they make better decisions.

Another important aspect of meditation is that it gives a feeling of contentment with very little stimulation. This is more important than ever in the modern world in which all of us can be so bombarded with sensory overload — work, advertising, TV, social media — and it becomes very easy to look for feeling good through wanting more and more stimulation as if the dial keeps getting turned up. Meditation allows the dial to be reset, finding the surprising way that stillness allows a sense of peaceful pleasure in itself. Then simple joys become more noticeable, whether the warmth of a summer's day, the beauty of a tree, or the joy of touch, awareness of the flow of energy. It can sound very clichéd but can be profound, as a respite from stress or a shift in life focus. Simple awareness of the breath is one path into mediation, moving more to a stillness of mind.

Stillness, peace and bliss

Stillness is one of those things that sounds almost simple in theory but is often very hard to find in practice.

One Indian sage, Sri H.W.L. Poonja, gave the example of how after people had worked hard for long periods to gain a particular prize, on achieving that prize they would often have an intense moment of peace and satisfaction. For that instant they stopped striving and were simply still. The mind paused for a moment. This stillness in itself allowed the sense of peace. Poonja was fond of saying that enlightenment only takes an instant, if we could just be still enough.[4]

On other levels, stillness is helpful in relaxation and healing, allowing the body's processes to work more deeply.

The breathing exercises in this book can lead to a greater stillness. One practice to achieve this is to do several rounds of slow full breathing (p. 67), then allow the breath to become passive, just noticing it without making any attempt to control or direct it, with simple mindful awareness of the breath. You can allow this awareness to spread through the body, just noticing any bodily sensations without trying to change anything, just simply being aware. Then just allow the mind to be still. You will find there are moments when the mind moves to this quiet, calm stillness. If any thoughts arise (which they are bound to now and then) simply notice the thoughts and let them pass, draw the awareness back to the breath and the body, again just noticing, moving more and more to the sense of stillness. The feeling is of allowing the mind to become empty rather than of making it be empty.

14

BREATHING WITH MOVEMENT

Breathing with fuller physical movement engages the body to extend the range of the breath and mobilize mind–body connections to relax, refresh or recharge.

People also tend to hold different patterns of stress in their bodies, through habitual holding of muscle tension. Simple stretches linked with the breath can help to release this, so has a refreshing and healing effect.

Make sure to go gently. Remember the focus is on the breath and gently having your awareness 'in' the body.

How to sit

The only really important thing about sitting for controlled breathing is to make sure you have a straight back — which is to say sitting tall and long through the spine, still allowing its natural gentle curves.

Everyone has probably seen some pictures of meditators sitting cross-legged on the floor. These types of poses are nice if you can do them, but are not for everyone. They originated in a time and place when people grew up sitting on the floor, so sitting cross-legged was natural. For most modern Westerners this takes a lot of practice, and it is not necessary. It is usually better to use a chair.

Sit forward so your sitting bones are almost on the edge of the chair. Have your thighs straight out and your feet flat on the floor. Try to find a chair that allows your thighs and calves to be close to a right angle and the thighs parallel to the floor, feet directly under your knees. You can place your hands on your thighs, or place them with one hand in the other, palms facing up, in your lap. A yoga variation is to rest the palms facing up on each thigh, with the thumb and first finger touching. This is called *jnana mudra* and gives a subtle sense of peacefulness and balance of energies.

Sitting like this you could do any of the breaths listed in the book.

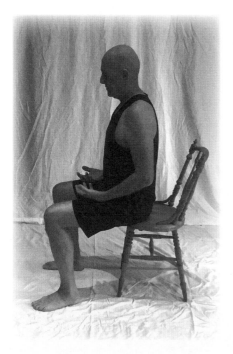 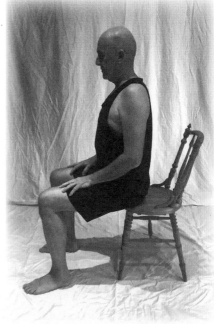

Seated breathing

The following breaths can be done individually or in combination. A simple, gentle way to refresh and feel alert and reenergized is to do several rounds of the spinal flexing breath, followed by the kelp breath followed by the twists. Then sit quietly for a few minutes doing a few rounds of controlled breathing — such as alternate nostril breathing (p. 80) or the full breath (p. 67). This simple sequence is a great break from office work.

SPINAL FLEXING BREATH

This breath gently opens the chest and mobilizes the spine. It is a great breath to do to stretch and refresh if you have been sitting at a desk for a while.

Sit tall and bring your arms up so that the upper arms stick out to the sides of the shoulders parallel to the floor, arms bent, with your forearms perpendicular to the floor, like 'stop signs'.

Take a breath in, then, moving slowly with the breath, on the exhalation bring the arms forward in front of you, rounding the back as you do so. Then breathing in, bring the arms slowly back to the starting position and slightly beyond it, arching the back gently, pulling the arms a bit behind the lines of the shoulders, keeping long through the spine and not collapsing.

Then continue, breathing out arms forward and rounding the back, breathing in arms back, gently flexing, allowing the movement to flow with the breath. This movement opens the chest, extends the range of the breath and mobilizes the spine. It is a gently energizing breath. Do three to seven breaths like this.

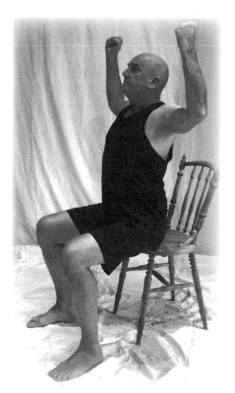 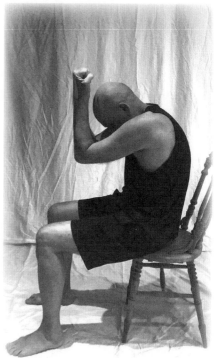

KELP BREATH

This breath mobilizes the spine and deepens the breath, as the movement of the body naturally enhances the exhalation from all the way down. It also encourages breathing to the back of the body, and is a great breath for calming and destressing.

Sit on a chair with your hands on your thighs just above your knees, knees hip width apart and your arms bent alongside your body. Breathing out, bend forward, rolling the spine so the torso moves forward with the belly first touching the thighs, then the chest comes onto the thighs, then the head comes down last. Going forward this way keeps the spine long as opposed to rounding the spine, so the head goes towards the knees with the back rounded. Feel the way that the movement extends and deepens the exhalation.

When breathing in, use the arms to support you and roll back up: first the lower back and then the upper back and head come up. Direct the breath more to the back of the body. This breath extends the exhalation and has a calming effect. Continue for three to seven slow breaths.

You might imagine the movement is like a strand of kelp flowing forward and backwards underneath the waves.

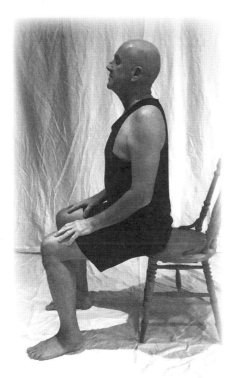
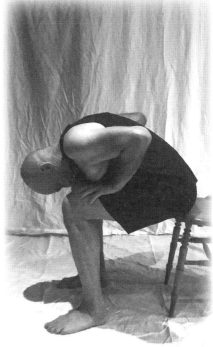

SEATED TWISTS

Begin by sitting tall with your hands just above the knees, then gently twist on an exhalation, taking your left hand behind you to hold the back or side of the chair and right hand in front over your left knee. Keeping tall, use the arms to gently aid you in twisting to look back over your left shoulder, trying to gently twist the whole length of the spine. Move slowly, twisting on the exhalation, then moving back to the centre on the inhalation. Then twist to the other side as you breathe out again.

Gently twisting like this brings life and energy to the spine and all the many nerves and organs connected to it, as well as a gentle wringing of the torso, which moves the passive fluids in the organs.

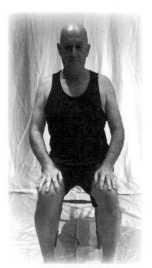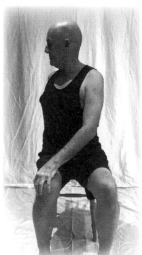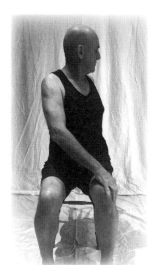

Standing breaths

These simple standing breaths open the back, the sides and front of the body. They can be done individually but are presented here as a sequence to discharge stress, feel grounded, open and energized. If you do them as a sequence, repeat each one three to seven times.

STANDING GROUNDING BREATH

Connecting with the energy of the Earth feels good whether you actually feel the flow of energy or just take it as a metaphor to visualize.

Stand with your feet hip width apart, knees bent, hands together in front of the navel or lower belly. As you breathe in, take the arms out to the sides and up until your hands come together again over your head. Take the arms down as you breathe out until your hands are again together in front of the lower belly. As you do this, imagine the energy of the Earth flowing up through your legs, through the base of your pelvis and into your body, filling the whole body. Breathe out any tension, imagining it flowing out down through the body, down through the legs and into the earth. You can picture the energy coming in as green or blue and the grey tensions flowing out. You might remember the *chi kung* belief that the Earth likes to recycle the stress like compost (see p. 106).

This breath also opens the side ribs, thus helping to extend the range of the breath.

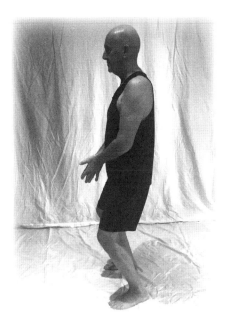
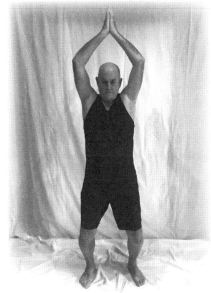

PELVIC BREATHING

The pelvic floor muscles are often neglected. They are important and provide a basis for the posture and a base for the breath.

When you engage the pelvic floor muscles on the exhalation there is a feeling of the flow of the breath extending and deepening. It aids and extends the gentle massage of the abdominal organs that occurs with diaphragmatic breathing, as well as being good for the organs of the pelvic area. Working this foundation brings a strength to the breath, and helps to direct energy upwards.

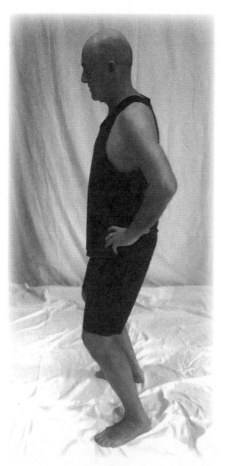

With your feet hip width apart and knees bent, take your hands to your hips, one hand on either side. As you breathe in, relax your hips and let them rock back a little, feeling as if you are breathing right to the middle of the pelvis. On the exhale squeeze the buttocks, the pelvic floor muscles, and the inner pelvic muscles, as if you are squeezing the air out right from the centre of the pelvis, letting the pelvis rock forward slightly. The hips will move forward a little as you do this, but only a little, the work is on the inside. On the inhalation relax the muscles and let the hips rock back a little. There is little external movement.

STANDING ARMPIT BREATH

This form opens the front of the body, so is energizing. It is a great pose in itself if you are feeling down and need a lift.

Stand tall with the legs straight, hands down by your sides, backs of your hands facing forwards. On the inhalation, raise your straight arms out to the front and then up, gently, until they are as far as is comfortable or until they are vertical above your head with the palms facing forwards. The action provides a gentle stretch to the entire front of the body — make sure to do it gently to begin, as it is stronger than it looks. Keep looking forward with the head steady, or if you have no neck problems gently look up as the arms reach above your head, and lower the head as the arms come down.

On the exhalation, lower the arms and hands to the starting position.

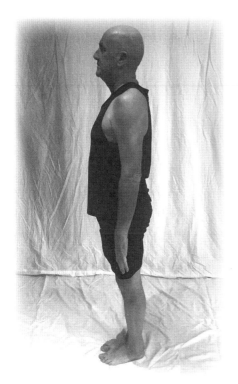
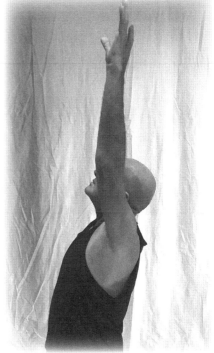

UPWARDS BREATH

This form opens the side ribs, extending the range of breathing. It also has an uplifting feeling of connecting to a higher purpose.

Standing tall, legs straight, take the hands down to the sides of the hips, palms facing outwards. As you breathe in take the arms up, taking them straight out from the sides of the body, going up until the hands are shoulder width apart, with the arms fully stretched above the head. Look straight ahead, or if you have no neck issues turn the head up to look at the hands as they go up. (You can imagine as you do this a sense of connecting with your higher potentials, whether this is in a spiritual sense or a metaphorical sense of your ideals and potentials.) On the out-breath, take the arms out to the sides and down.

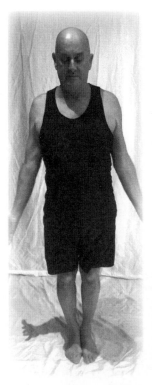
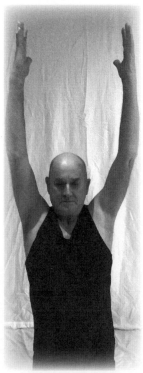
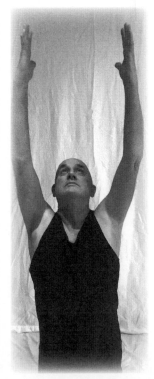

STANDING FULL BREATH

This form uses conscious alignment to bring strength and balance. Although you are not moving, this pose is active as you take your awareness and gentle adjustments through the body. This is the classic mountain pose of yoga (known as *tadasana*).

First, be aware of your feet on the ground, then your calves, then pull the kneecaps up as you engage the quadriceps in the front of the thighs. Tuck your tail in a little as you gently engage the glutes (buttocks). Draw the belly in, gently engaging the abdominals as if you were about to put on a pair of tight jeans. Open the shoulders wide, engaging the muscles between the shoulder blades and feel that this slightly opens the upper chest. Have the arms down by the sides, stretched out with the fingers apart as if a flow of energy is going through them. Feel as if the head is lifted up by a string, with the back of the neck long and the chin very slightly tucked in. Hold this awareness as best you can as you breathe — breathing down the back of the body, breathing up the back all the way from the pelvic bowl, ending with the breath coming forward to the front of the upper chest.

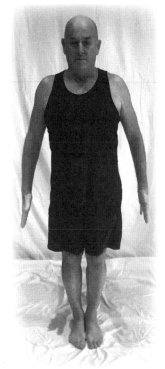

Exhale in reverse: first from the upper chest then drawing in the ribs, then the belly. At the end of the exhalation, draw the pelvic muscles gently in, up and towards the back. As you breathe in again, don't completely let go; hold a gentle firmness of the muscles as you draw the breath again down the back of the body.

There is a lot of direction here, but the main thing is to try to bring awareness and activation to the whole body. The pose has a strength and power to it, like the mountain after which it is named.

After a few breaths like this, you can either simply finish or do the following:

Set your intention or goal for the day, saying it gently to yourself or picturing it. When the mind is calm, as it usually is after this stretching and breathing, setting intentions tends to have a special power. This can be understood in different ways, whether more scientifically in terms of the brainwave frequencies which are predominant in these calm focused states, or more spiritually in terms of being more open at these times to being in touch with a 'higher self'.

If you are spiritually inclined it is a good time to offer a prayer or to ask for such guidance or support as you might seek.

The end of such a sequence is a good time for meditation, as you have stretched and released tension. You can then sit and do a few controlled breaths and move into meditation, such as a gentle focus on the passive breath.

Breathing on the floor

The following are breath forms to do on the floor. As long as you have a clean floor, you don't need any equipment, though a yoga mat, rug or simple fabric (like a sarong) to cover the floor are all good options.

It is best to take off your shoes and socks, and be wearing something that allows movement, such as shorts or tights.

CHILD'S POSE: RELEASING

This pose is great to relax and calm. It directs the breath naturally to the back of the body and engenders a sense of surrender.

Kneel down and take your knees apart, a little wider than hip width, while having the big toes touching, then roll forward so your forehead comes to the floor, taking your arms and hands gently forward and keeping the arms slightly or more fully bent so there is no strain (if you don't have this range of movement then comfortably take your elbows to the floor as you lean forward). Feel that the breath moves more to the back of the body and gently allow yourself to let go of any tension, allowing the back to soften and slowly extend. Stay here for several slow breaths.

You will probably notice the body release after a few breaths and you can inch your arms and head forward a little as you release into the pose. Another variation is to take your hands back beside your feet. Once you have finished, come onto your hands and knees before getting up.

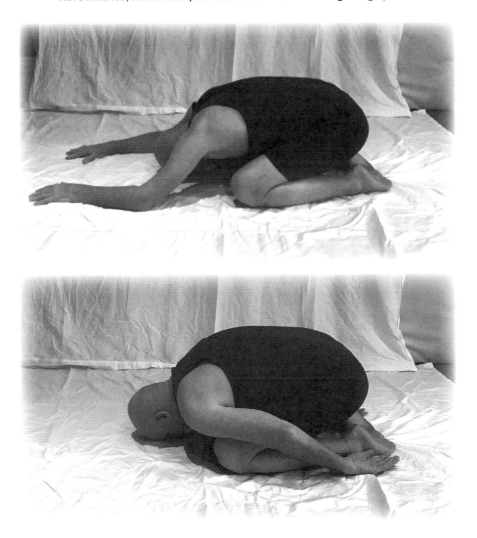

CAT/COW BREATHING

This simple stretch is a good way to gently mobilize the spine and deepen the breath.

Come onto your hands and knees on the floor. Your knees should be directly below your hips, and your hands directly below your shoulders.

On the exhalation round your back, bringing your head and hips towards each other. On the inhalation concave your back, lifting the head and hips higher. Move slowly and focus on deepening the breath, especially to exhale fully. Try to deepen awareness with each movement. Draw the belly in on the exhalation, feeling as if the muscles work in a wave until you feel as if you are breathing out all the way from the pelvic floor.

Do seven or more breaths like this.

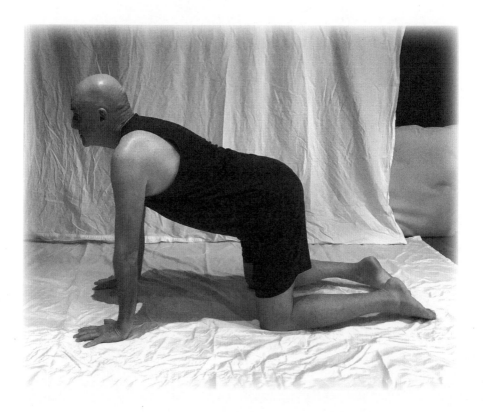

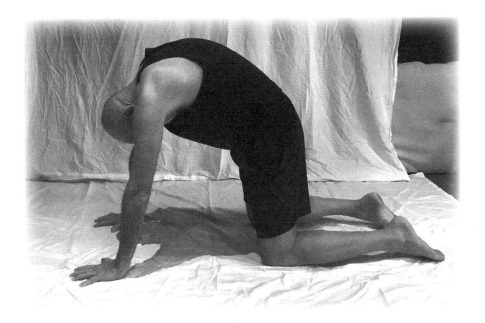

Child's pose followed by some cat/cow stretching gives a great release then a gentle energizing, linked with a sense of really 'being in the body'.

If you want more you could begin with these, then do the standing sequence (pp. 164–70).

If you just want to deeply relax then after child's pose and cat/cow you could just lie on your back for a few minutes.

RELAXATION

Deep relaxation has huge benefits for mind and body, and just lying still is a deceptively good practice, especially after some gentle movements to release any tensions. Yoga practitioners will recognize this as *savasana* or 'corpse pose'.

Lie on your back, with your feet several inches apart (as feels comfortable). You might like a small pillow under your head — see what feels comfortable for you. Stretch out and if you have any lower back issues, you can keep your knees bent, with feet on the floor, or place a pillow or rolled up blanket under your knees; otherwise stretch the legs out so the body is long. Allow the feet to fall out to the sides. Have the arms down and a few inches out from the side of the body, palms facing up, which opens the chest slightly and opens the breathing more.

Allow yourself to become still. If your mind wanders bring it back to awareness of the breath, then allow awareness of the body sensations, then as much as you can, just let go.

After a few minutes gently roll to your right-hand side and gradually come back up to sitting. Allow some time to sit, and if you'd like, add some breathing or meditation before getting up and going back to your day.

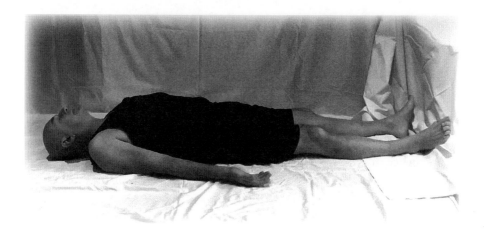

15

SUBTLE ENERGIES

Purposeful breathing is a central part of many Eastern traditions, including practices for health and healing, spiritual enlightenment and martial arts. In older times some of these techniques were closely guarded secrets, which often required the trainee to undergo an initiation before being taught. By contrast, in contemporary times myriad different techniques can be found just by clicking on the internet, though, like everything else on the internet, there can be trash as well as treasure.

While introductory levels of yoga and martial arts may focus just on physical disciplines, advanced levels have the common feature of focusing on ways to expand, control and direct energy.

This idea of expanding energy can seem odd in the West, but the idea of an energy body is basic to both Chinese and Indian medical and spiritual traditions. Acupuncture is based on the map of energy channels accepted in Chinese medicine. It is widely accepted in the West, as evidenced by the number of people who use such treatments and its acceptance by health insurance funds. Many Western doctors now use acupuncture, even though there is no Western medical explanation for why it might work. Chinese medicine provides a precise map of energy channels, or meridians, and health problems occur if the channels become 'blocked' or if the flow of energy through them is imbalanced. The acupuncture needles placed at specific points in these channels allow the energy to flow more freely and to increase or decrease the flow in different channels. This flow of energy might also be directed through meditational practice or through disciplines such as tai chi and advanced yoga.

Day-to-day experiences related to this energy body might be the 'charge' we feel when we are attracted to someone. The connection we feel with people can have diverse forms. Many people experience something like an energy flow between them which is not fully explained by emotional terms or shared ideas alone.

Purposeful breathing can be used to build and direct energy, and practising controlled breathing develops a subtlety of awareness that helps in turn to develop awareness of the life energy.

Pranayama

Pranayama is the yogic science of the breath. The word *pranayama* is made up of two Sanskrit words: *prana*, which means the energy of the breath, and *yama*, which means control. This implies that *pranayama* is the control of the breath.

Prana sometimes refers specifically to the energy of the breath, and sometimes it is used to refer to the body's energies as a whole: 'life energy' in general. In its broader meaning, *prana* can be seen to be linked with the word *ayama*, which means expansion. In this meaning, *pranayama* is a science and art of expanding energy, creating more vitality in the body.

There are many forms of breathing linked with *pranayama*,[1] most of which are best learnt under the supervision of a qualified teacher, but others can be taught here and have informed many of the practices in this book, such as an emphasis on extending the exhalation for calming, the three-part breath to energize (p. 124) or alternate nostril breathing (p. 80).

A further practice is the following, which extends on the one described on p. 75.

EXTENDED 1:2 BREATH

Sit with a straight back, either cross-legged or on a chair.

The exhalation for this breath is twice as long as the inhalation, but never force anything or strain, so initially practice with inhalation and exhalation the same length. Then as you get used to it, slowly extend the exhalation.

For the first breath just breathe in fully, then on the exhalation allow the breath to passively release, relaxing and allowing the natural elasticity of the lungs to draw back in and the diaphragm to rise. Then, when you are almost at the end of the passive exhalation, draw in the abdomen, especially feeling as if the lower belly (from where it attaches just above the pubic bone) draws backwards. When most of that air is expelled draw the pelvic floor in and up, and finally pull the anus in and tilt it up and backwards. In yoga terms this helps the energy ascend, but for everyday purposes you can feel it extends the last of the exhalation.

Then as you inhale, don't release the abdominal muscles much but feel the breath begin at the back of the body so the back of the diaphragm engages, then allowing the side ribs to open and finally draw the air to the front of the upper chest.

These aspects are best done in a ratio — so if the total count is in for eight and out for sixteen, you would breathe in to the diaphragm (directed to the back of the diaphragm) for four, expand the side ribs for two and the upper chest for two. Then breathe out passively for eight, drawing in the lower abdomen for four, pelvic floor for two, and drawing up the perineum and anus for two. It takes a while to get the ratios right but eventually the aim is that the exhalation is twice the length of the inhalation.

The ratio of 1:2 means you are getting really full breaths without hyperventilating, and the longer exhalation has a calming effect. Involving the anus will feel very weird to some people but with a little practice you can feel the sense of energy ascending, and the practice feels at once uplifting, energizing and very calm.

Extensions

It would seem remiss in a section on *pranayama* not to include the 'victorious breath' or *ujjayi*.

Ujjayi breathing is popular in many yoga classes and involves gently partially closing the glottis, so that a deep whispering sound is heard. The usual way to learn it is to imagine you are going to fog up a window on a cold day. This sound as you breathe out is produced by the partial closure of the glottis. This partial closure is kept while breathing through the nose and through both the inhalation and exhalation. Another way it is taught is to whisper, then hold the whisper sound as you breathe in and out through the nose. The sound is soft and subtle. This breath has a very interiorizing effect, to take you inside, and it helps hear the breath so as to aid in it being very smooth and even. While mentioned here, it is best learnt from a teacher, and please stop if you try it and feel any discomfort.

Another helpful *pranayama* practice is to allow the natural pauses between the inhalation and exhalation, and also the pause after exhalation. Just allowing and noticing these has a deep sense of peace about it, as there is often a suspension of thought concomitant with the suspension of breath.

Pranayama also often involves conscious breath holding. The key with this is to keep it gentle and never strain (breath holding can cause blood pressure to rise). One popular practice is 'square breathing' — breathing in for a count of four, hold for four, out for four and suspend the breath for four. I personally like to often use a breathing practice of in for four, hold for four, out for eight and hold out for four.

Rather than specifically counting the holds, I recommend if you are interested in this to just allow a pause at the end of the in-breath and a pause at the end of the out-breath. Pausing after the exhalation has a deep sense of peacefulness about it. This type of breathing fully oxygenates the system but the pauses also ensures that the carbon dioxide levels remain well balanced, so that the blood vessels are dilated, which is good for brain and body.

Pranayama also includes some vigorous practices but these are best done under expert guidance.

Choosing where to centre

Both *pranayama* and *chi kung* (see p. 48) have a focus on circulating energy through the energy centres of the body.

The yogic traditions focus mostly on drawing energy up the spine, through the chakras. *Chi kung* draws energy from the Earth and the cosmos and circulates it in different channels around the body.[2] Full outlines of these practices would be entire books in themselves, but a simple practice is to imagine the energy of the breath ascending from the base of the spine, up the spine to the crown of the head on the in-breath, and descending back down on the out-breath. This can help to make sure energy is not blocked.

This allows us to choose where to centre out energies. This can be in the *hara* or lower *tan tien* as described on p. 104, or in the heart. Centring in the *hara* gives a sense of strength that is very helpful if you are facing challenges. Centring in the higher energy centres is done in meditation and with some guidance.

For everyday focus, a great way to centre is in the heart.

Breathing to fill the heart

I often finish my own yoga practice with centring in the heart, and some yoga schools have the tradition of finishing a class by focusing on the heart and chanting 'om, shanti, shanti, shanti', with 'shanti' meaning a sense of peace and intention of love to all sentient beings. Although we may want to shift energies at different times for different purposes, being centred in the heart opens a sense of joy and connection with other people and the world around us.

The heart has long been seen in many traditions as the centre of love and emotion. Recent science has shown it is not simply a pump, but also has a nerve centre that in many ways is its own brain — the cardiac plexus — and also acts a gland, releasing hormones as part of the endocrine system.

As well as the literal physical organ, the energetic heart is the centre of love in Western art and the energy centre of Eastern traditions. Imagine this as in line with the actual heart or a little higher in the chest. Religious pictures of the radiant heart of Jesus are a perfect illustration of this, but of course it does not need to be linked to any religious tradition.

HEART-CENTRED BREATH

This is a beautiful breath to include as the last of many in this book.

First place one or both of your hands on your upper chest, above your physical heart area. Consciously breathe to the energetic heart area and visualize it shining and filling the whole chest area. As you breathe in, imagine the energy of the breath going to this area. As you breathe out, allow the energy to expand through you.

This breath should be gentle, not forceful. Allow and imagine the heart area to become radiant. Let it fill you. Smile to it. Let the energy spread through your body. If you like, let the energy flow out beyond you, to fill the area around you, then draw it back in before you finish, so it is centred in the upper chest area.

All of us have a capacity for radiance and this is a great breath for allowing your light to shine.

Play

This book has listed many different techniques, and many types of breathing for specific purposes, but every individual will be a bit different and it is important to explore what feels right for you. Some of the breaths may produce different effects for each us. So when trying a few of the breaths, tune in to how they work for you personally.

The important thing here is to be invited to play with the different styles of breathing — it is not about memorizing formulas, but rather being more deeply in touch with your own body.

- **How does it feel for you if you breathe low, middle or high?**
- **How does it feel to breathe through the nose, not the mouth, and if you breathe through the mouth how can you change the shape of it to slow, speed up or channel the breath?**
- **Which styles of breathing feel good?**
- **Which ones feel uplifting, which ones energizing, which ones calming?**
- **How does your breathing change with different moods?**

Focusing on the breath can be part of developing deeper awareness of embodied responses, greater interoception. We humans are not just thought-clouds floating in space; all of our thoughts, emotions and actions are deeply embodied. Being more aware of the breath allows us greater awareness on several levels, as breath reflects mood, tension, calm or agitation. The breath is like a great portable biofeedback machine, reflecting both more awareness and more control over mood.

Play with the different styles of breathing and notice your own personal responses. Here is a shortlist of ones to try from time to time:

- **the five or six per minute breath ('breaths per minute')**
- **high or low or full**
- **diaphragmatic breathing**
- **circular breathing**
- **controlled exhalation versus passive exhalation**
- **alternate nostril**
- **slow or muscular**
- **front, centre or back.**

Not every variation will produce a discernible difference, but some will and there are many variations to play with. The more you practise, the more subtle your awareness becomes.

There are a huge number of possible permutations for different breathing styles. All of them can be combined — you can, for example, breathe to the back of the chest, with a long exhalation, with no holding, slowly, through the nose, etc. I'm not suggesting you become obsessive, but play with a few.

Everybody is a bit different and if you become more aware of how a few purposeful breaths work for you, that awareness is more important than following any set formula.

CONCLUSION: EVERYDAY INSPIRATION

Historically, breath and spirit were often interlinked. Inspiration meant not just breathing in air, but being *in-spirited*, having the spirit filled and lifted. This book has aimed to explore and renew many of these links between breath and spirit, showing the links between different patterns of breathing and different emotional states, the ways that states of mind are intertwined with styles of breath, mapping out many of the myriad ways breath and body interlink and more broadly how our spirits can be deflated or uplifted by these very literal and embodied forms of inspiration and expiration.

The breath is arguably the most powerful and immediate of our mind–body links, and changing the style of breathing is an effective way to change mental states and modes of being. A few purposeful breaths can enable anyone to feel calmer, stronger and more centred. Of course, if you are anxious, a few breaths may not take away the causes of your anxiety, but it will help you face them in a manner that feels more empowered.

A few purposeful breaths can give a pause to reset your mind and enhance your energy. They can help you feel better in the short term and in the longer term enhance your health by bringing your systems into balance.

I hope that in reading this book you may have become aware that you are probably already an expert in important skills you may not have known you had, and that the book has given you further skills and ways to refine and extend your pre-existing ones.

Simple breathing can be a source of strength, stability and focus; a pathway into deeper awareness of the body and our many mind–body connections; and a simple, powerful way to find stillness, peace and joy amidst the bustle and complexities of modern life.

APPENDIX:
THE BREATHING STYLES

ACKNOWLEDGMENTS

Thanks to the many friends and colleagues who have supported me in this endeavour. Special thanks to my many clients who have engaged in the practices described in the book.

I would also especially like to acknowledge and thank Colleen Lewig and Vicki McCoy for supporting the many breathing, yoga and meditation classes that I have run over the years at the University of Adelaide; Catherine Leahy, Katy Perisic, Felicity Chapman and Michael Beilby for comments on earlier drafts of the manuscript; Eero Riikonen, Michael Lennon and Leonie Nowland for encouragement and inspiration; Rob Hall for his enthusiasm; and Mark O'Donoghue for our many finely detailed conversations on meditation and *pranayama*.

REFERENCES

Ackerman, C. 2019, 'The 23 amazing health benefits of mindfulness for body and brain', https://positivepsychologyprogram.com/benefits-of-mindfulness/

Benson, H. with Klipper M.Z. 1976, *The Relaxation Response*, HarperCollins, New York.

Bernadi, L. et al. 2001, 'Modulatory effects of respiration', *Autonomic Neuroscience* 90: pp. 47–56.

Brouillard C. et al. 2016, 'Long-lasting Bradypnea by repeated social defeat', *American Journal of Physiology-Regulatory, Integrative and Comparative Physiology* 311, R352–64.

Brown, R.P. and Gerbarg, P.L. 2012, *The Healing Power of the Breath*, Shambala Publications, Boston.

Burke, A. and Marconett, S. 2008, The role of breath in Yogic traditions: Alternate nostril breathing, *Biofeedback* 36, (2), pp. 67-69.

Byrne, R. 2006, *The Secret*, Atria, New York.

Calais-Germain, B. 2006, *Anatomy of Breathing*, Eastland Press, Seattle.

Calasso, R. 1994, *The Marriage of Cadmus and Harmony*, Vintage Books, New York.

Chaitow, L., Bradley D. and Gilbert, C. 2014, *Recognizing and Treating Breathing Disorders: A multidisciplinary approach*, 2nd ed., Elsevier, London.

Chia, M. 1983, *Awaken Healing Energy Through the Tao*, Aurora Press, Santa Fe.

Chia, M. 1993, *Awaken Healing Light of the Tao*, Healing Tao Books, Huntington.

Crum, A. Akinola, M., Martin, A. and Fath, S. 2017, 'The role of stress mindset in shaping cognitive, emotional, and physiological responses to challenging and threatening stress', *Anxiety, Stress, Coping*, 30(4): pp. 379–95.

Csikszentmihalyi, M. 1992, *Flow: The psychology of happiness*, Harper and Row, New York.

Csikszentmihalyi, M. 1996, *Creativity: Flow and the psychology of discovery and invention*, Harper Perennial, New York.

De Shazer, S. 1985, *Keys to Solution in Brief Therapy*, W.W. Norton, New York.

Dickerson, H. 'Nitric oxide and mouth breathing', https://www.lviglobal.com/wp-content/uploads/2017/06/NitricOxideMouthBreathing.pdf

Ehrmann. W. 2017, *Coherent Breathing: Aligning breath and heart*, Tao de in Kamphausen Mediengruppe GmbH, Bielefeld.

Elliott, S. with Edmunson, D. 2006, *The New Science of the Breath*, 2nd ed. Coherence Press, Allen, TA.

Emerson, D. 2015, Tr*auma-sensitive Yoga in Therapy: Bringing the body into treatment*, W.W. Norton, New York.

Emerson, D. and Hopper, E. 2011, *Overcoming Trauma Through Yoga: Reclaiming your body*, North Atlantic Books, Berkeley.

Fowler, Clare, J. 2003, 'Visceral sensory neuroscience: Interoception' *Brain*, 126: (6), pp. 1505–1506.

Fried, R. 1990, *The Breath Connection*, Plenum Press, New York.

Fried, R. 1999, *Breathe Well, Be Well: A program to relieve stress, anxiety, asthma, hypertension, migraine, and other disorders for better health*, Wiley, New York.

Fried, R. 2013, *The Psychology and Physiology of Breathing in Behavioral Medicine, Clinical Psychology, and Psychiatry*, Springer Science & Business Media, New York.

Gardner H. 2006, *Multiple Intelligences: New horizons in theory and practice*, Basic Books, New York.

Goleman, D. 1995, *Emotional Intelligence: Why it can matter more than IQ*, Bantam Books, New York.

Graham, T. 2014, *Relief from Snoring and Sleep Apnoea*, Penguin, Melbourne.

Graham, T. 2017, *Relief from Anxiety and Panic by Changing How You Breathe*, BreatheAbility Publications.

Grof, S. and Grof, C. 2010, *Holotropic Breathwork*, SUNY Press, New York.

Iovine, J. 1993, *Kirlian Photography: A hands-on guide*, McGraw-Hill, New York.

Iyengar, B.K.S. 1981, *Light on Pranayama*, Aquarian Press, London.

Kabat-Zinn, J. 2013, *Full Catastrophe Living: How to cope with stress, pain and illness using mindfulness meditation*, Bantam Books, New York.

Keller, A. et al. 2011, 'Does the perception that stress affects health matter? The association with health and mortality', *Health Psychology*, 31 (5) pp. 677–84.

Kozlowska, K., Walker, P., McLean, L. and Carrive, P. 2015, 'Fear and the defensive cascade: Clinical implications and management', *Harvard Review of Psychiatry*, 23(4), pp. 263–87.

Lalande, L., King, R., Bambling, M. and Schweitzer R.D. 2016, 'Guided respiration mindfulness therapy: Development and evaluation of a brief therapist training program', *Journal of Contemporary Psychotherapy*, 46(2), pp. 107–16.

Maehle, G. 2012, *Pranayama: The breath of yoga*, Kaivalya Publications, Innaloo City, Western Australia.

McConnell, A. 2011, *Breathe Strong Perform Better*, Human Kinetics, Leeds.

McGonigal, K. 2015, *The Upside of Stress*, Vermillion, London.

Miller. A.H. and Raison C.L. 2016, 'The role of inflammation in depression: From evolutionary imperative to modern treatment target', *Nature Reviews Immunology*, 16, pp. 22–34.

Peterson C. and Seligman M. 2004, *Character Strengths and Virtues: A handbook and classification*, Oxford University Press, Oxford.

Poonja H.W.L. 1995, *The Truth Is*, Yudishatara, Lucknow.

Porges, S.W. 2011, *The Polyvagal Theory: Neurophysiological foundations of emotions, attachment, communication, and self-regulation*, W.W. Norton, New York.

Porges, S.W. 2017, *The Pocket Guide to The Polyvagal Theory: The transformative power of feeling safe*, Norton, New York.

Rakhimov, A. 2014, *Normal Breathing: The key to vital health*, Createspace Independent Publishing Platform.

Russo, M.A., Santarelli D.M. and O'Rourke D. 2017, 'The physiological effects of slow breathing in the healthy human', *Breathe*, 13(4), pp. 298–309.

Saraswati, Swami Niranjanananda. 2009, *Pranan and Pranayama*, Yoga Publications Trust, Bihar.

Siegel, D. 2007, *The Mindful Brain: Reflection and attunement in the cultivation of wellbeing*, Norton, New York.

Sikter, A., Rihmer, Z. and de Guevara, R. 2017, 'New aspects in the patho-mechanism of diseases of civilization, particularly psychosomatic disorders. Part 1: Theoretical background of a hypothesis', *Neuropsychopharmacologia Hungaria* XIX , (95–104), pp. 159–69.

Simpkins C.A. and Simpkins A.M. 2010, *Neuro-hypnosis: Using self-hypnosis to activate the brain for change*, Norton, New York.

Telles, S. and Nilkamal, S. 2014, 'A review of the use of yoga in breathing dis-orders', in Chaitow, L., Bradley, D. and Gilbert C., *Recognizing and Treating Breathing Disorders: A multidisciplinary approach*, 2nd ed. Elsevier, London.

Tripathi, P. 2007, 'Nitric oxide and immune response', *Indian J Biochemistry and Biophysiology*, 44(5), pp. 310–19.

Watzlawick, P., Weakland, J. and Fisch, R. 1974, *Change: Principles of problem formation and problem resolution*, W.W. Norton, New York.

Weintraub, A. 2004, *Yoga for Depression*, Broadway Books, New York.

Wolinsky, S. 1991, *Trances People Live*, Bramble Books, Falls Village CT.

Yerkes, R.M. and Dodson J. D. 1908, 'The relation of strength of stimulus to rapidity of habit-formation', *Journal of Comparative Neurology and Psychology*, 18, pp. 459–82.

Yogi Ramacharaka, 1904, *Science of Breath: A complete manual of the Oriental breathing philosphy of physical, mental, psychic and spiritual development*, Yogi Publication Society, Chicago.

Zaccaro A. et al. 2018, 'How breath-control can change your life: A systematic review on psycho-physiological correlates of slow breathing', *Frontiers in Human Neuroscience*, 12, p. 353.

ENDNOTES

Chapter 2: Breathing awareness

1. Lundberg J.O. et al. 1995, 'High nitric oxide production in human paranasal sinuses', *Nat Med*, 1, pp. 370–3.
2. Zaccaro A. et al. 2018, 'How breath-control can change your life: A systematic review on psycho-physiological correlates of slow breathing', *Frontiers in Human Neuroscience*, 12, p. 353.
3. Yogi Ramacharaka. 1904, *Science of Breath: A complete manual of the Oriental breathing philosophy of physical, mental, psychic and spiritual development*, Yogi Publication Society, Chicago, pp. 27, 29.

Chapter 3: Key mechanisms

1. I have drawn here on the books and training by Tess Graham, especially Graham, T. 2017, *Relief from Anxiety and Panic by Changing How You Breathe*, BreatheAbility Publications, p. 42.
2. Sikter, A., Rihmer, Z. and de Guevara, R. 2017, 'New aspects in the pathomechanism of diseases of civilization, particularly psychosomatic disorders', in *Neuropsychopharmacologia Hungaria*, Part One: June,19 (2), pp. 95–105 and Part Two: November 19(3), pp. 159–69.
3. Lundberg J.O. et al. 1995.
4. I have drawn here from the excellent summary by Heidi Dickerson at https://www.lviglobal.com/wp-content/uploads/2017/06/ NitricOxideMouthBreathing.pdf and also Tripathi, P. 2007, 'Nitric oxide and immune response', *Indian J Biochemistry and Biophysiology*, October, 44(5), pp. 310–19.
5. This list is drawn from presentations given by Sue Hetzel to the Graduate Program in Counselling and Psychotherapy, University of Adelaide, 12 September 2013.
6. Porges, S.W. 2011, *The Polyvagal Theory: Neurophysiological foundations of emotions, attachment, communication, and self-regulation*, W.W. Norton, New York, or as an introductory guide: Porges, S.W. 2017, *The Pocket Guide to The Polyvagal Theory: The transformative power of feeling safe*, Norton, New York.

7. Gardner H. 2006, *Multiple Intelligences: New horizons in theory and practice*, Basic Books, New York; Goleman, D. 1995, *Emotional Intelligence: Why it can matter more than IQ*, Bantam Books, New York.
8. I was drawn to this definition quoted in Emerson, D. 2015, T*rauma-sensitive Yoga in Therapy: Bringing the body into treatment*, W.W. Norton, New York. The original reference is Fowler, Clare, J. 2003, 'Visceral sensory neuroscience: Interoception', *Brain*, 126 (6), pp. 1505–6.
9. Quoted in Ehrmann, W. 2017, *Coherent Breathing: Aligning breath and heart*, Tao de in Kamphausen Mediengruppe GmbH, Bielefeld, p. 30.
10. From Ehrmann, W. 2017, p. 43.
11. A good overview of this is in Brown, R.P. and Gerberg, P.L. 2012, *The Healing Power of the Breath*, Shambala Publications, Boston.
12. The technique involves having an object connected to a high voltage source while on a photographic plate, and is attributed to the Russian Semyon Kirlian. See Iovine, J. 1993, *Kirlian Photography: A hands-on guide*, McGraw-Hill, New York, and a good overview, including sample photographs, is provided on Wikipedia: https://en.wikipedia.org/wiki/Kirlian_photography

Chapter 4: Problem breathing
1. Fried, R. 2013, *The Psychology and Physiology of Breathing in Behavioral Medicine, Clinical Psychology, and Psychiatry*, Springer Science & Business Media; Fried, R. 1990, *The Breath Connection*, Plenum Press, New York; Fried, R. 1999, *Breathe Well, Be Well: A program to relieve stress, anxiety, asthma, hypertension, migraine, and other disorders for better health*, Wiley, New York.
2. This list was identified in 1978 by Missri and Alexander and quoted in Fried, 1990.
3. Chaitow, L., Bradley D. and Gilbert, C. 2014, *Recognizing and Treating Breathing Disorders: A multidisciplinary approach*, 2nd ed. Elsevier, London.
4. Graham, T. 2014, *Relief from Snoring and Sleep Apnoea*, Penguin, Melbourne.
5. Sikter, A., Rihmer, Z. and de Guevara, R. 2017, 'New aspects in the pathomechanism of diseases of civilization, particularly psychosomatic disorders. Parts 1 and 2' in *Neuropsychopharmacologia Hungaria*, Jun; 19(2), pp. 95–105 and see also Kozlowska, K., Walker, P., McLean, L. and Carrive, P. 2015, 'Fear and the defensive cascade: Clinical implications and management', *Harvard Review of Psychiatry*, 23(4), pp. 263–28.

6. Brouillard, C. et al. 2016, 'Long-lasting bradypnea by repeated social defeat', *American Journal of Physiology-Regulatory, Integrative and Comparative Physiology*, 311, R352–64.
7. Sikter, A. Rihmer, Z. and de Guevara, R. 2017.

Chapter 6: Breathing styles and basic techniques

1. Emerson, D. and Hopper, E. 2011, *Overcoming Trauma Through Yoga: Reclaiming your body*, North Atlantic Books, Berkeley.
2. There are choices here for the direction of the movement, whether you breathe in and out from the lower lungs progressing to the top, or in and out from the top first and progressing down. Some people call this 'bucket' breathing or 'balloon' breathing, depending whether you fill and empty from the bottom or the top. Although subtle, there is a difference in that when the air is held longer in the upper lungs it tends to induce a more 'heady' feeling, and when held in the lower lungs longer, it tends to feel more calm and 'in the body'.
3. Maximum heart rate variability is maximized at about six breaths per minute, research by Bernadi, L. et al. 2001 and others, as cited in Russo, M.A., Santarelli D.M. and O'Rourke D. 2017, 'The physiological effects of slow breathing in the healthy human', *Breathe*, 13(4), pp. 298–309.
4. Elliott, S. with Edmunson, D. 2006, *The New Science of the Breath*, 2nd ed. Coherence Press, Allen, TX, p. 34.
5. Brown, R. P. and Gerberg, P.L. 2012 *The Healing Power of the Breath* Shambala Publications, Boston.
6. Zaccaro, A. et al. 2018.
7. 'Breatheability' training seminar with Tess Graham, 2017.
8. Weinstraub, A. 2004, *Yoga for Depression*, Broadway Books, New York, p. 130.
9. Burke, A. and Marconett, S. 2008, 'The role of breath in yogic traditions: Alternate nostril breathing', *Biofeedback*, 36 (2), pp. 67–9.
10. Quoted in Weinstraub, A. 2004, p. 136.
11. Wolinsky, S. 1991, *Trances People Live*, Bramble Books, Falls Village, CT.

Chapter 7: Stop, Breathe, Refocus

1. Peterson C. and Seligman M. 2004 *Character Strengths and Virtues: A Handbook and Classification*, Oxford University Press, Oxford.
2. Peterson C. and Seligman M. 2004.

Chapter 8: Managing and transforming stress

1. Yerkes, R.M. and Dodson J. D. 1908, 'The relation of strength of stimulus to rapidity of habit-formation', *Journal of Comparative Neurology and Psychology*, 18: pp. 459–82.
2. Recent research on the potential benefits of stress have been well collated by Kelly McGonigal in her book *The Upside of Stress*. She also has a very entertaining TED talk: https://www.ted.com/talks/kelly_mcgonigal_how_to_make_stress_your_friend?language=en
3. McGonigal, K. 2015, *The Upside of Stress*, Vermillion, London, p. 9.
4. This research is also outlined in McGonigal's book *The Upside of Stress*.

Chapter 9: Anxiety, trauma and depression

1. See Emerson, D. and Hopper, E. 2011, *Overcoming Trauma Through Yoga: Reclaiming your body*, North Atlantic Books, Berkeley; and Emerson, D. 2015, Tr*auma-sensitive Yoga in Therapy: Bringing the body into treatment*, W.W. Norton, New York.
2. See, for example, Miller, A.H. and Raison, C.L. 2016, 'The role of inflammation in depression: From evolutionary imperative to modern treatment target', *Nature Reviews Immunology*, 16, pp. 22–34.

Chapter 10: Enhancing energy

1. See, for example, Utay, J. and Miller, M. 2006, 'Guided imagery as an effective therapeutic technique: A brief review of its history and efficacy research', *Journal of Instructional Psychology*, 33 (1), pp. 40–3.
2. Especially Byrne, R. 2006, *The Secret*, Atria Books New York.

Chapter 11: Health and physical goals

1. Rakhimov, A. 2014, *Normal Breathing: The key to vital health*, Createspace Independent Publishing Platform.
2. Sundar Balasuramanian presents his research on 'The science of yogic breathing': https://www.youtube.com/watch?v=aIfwbEvXtwo
3. Russo, M.A., Santarelli D.M. and O'Rourke D. 2017.
4. See also Zaccaro, A. et al. 2018.
5. Especially Kabat-Zinn, J. 2013, *Full Catastrophe Living: How to cope with stress, pain and illness using mindfulness meditation*, Bantam Books, New York.
6. See McConnell, A. 2011, *Breathe Strong, Perform Better*, Human Kinetics Books, Leeds.

Chapter 12: Happiness, inspiration, creativity
1. Csikszentmihalyi, M. 1996, *Creativity: Flow and the psychology of discovery and invention*, Harper Perennial, New York, p. 104.
2. Csikszentmihalyi, M. 1992, *Flow: The psychology of happiness*, Harper and Row, New York.

Chapter 13: Breathing as a means of meditation
1. There is now a large number of books on mindfulness. One leading proponent is Dan Siegel, author of *The Mindful Brain: Reflection and attunement in the cultivation of wellbeing*, Norton, New York. A good introductory overview of this research can be found at https://positivepsychologyprogram.com/benefits-of-mindfulness/
2. Benson, H. with Klipper, M.Z. 1976, *The Relaxation Response*, HarperCollins New York.
3. Telles, S. and Nilkamal, S. 2014, 'A review of the use of yoga in breathing disorders' in Chaitow, L., Bradley, D. and Gilbert C. 2014, *Recognizing and Treating Breathing Disorders: A multidisciplinary approach*, 2nd ed. Elsevier, London.
4. Poonja, H.W.L. 1995, *The Truth Is*, Yudishatara, Lucknow.

Chapter 15: Subtle Energies
1. For further reading on the breadth and precision of these breathing techniques, see Saraswati, Swami Niranjanananda. 2009, 2016, *Prana and Pranayama*, Yoga Publications Trust, Bihar; or Iyengar, B. K. S. 1981, 1992, *Light on Pranayama*, Aquarian Press, London.
2. See, for example, Mantak Chia's books: Chia, M. 1983, *Awaken Healing Energy Through the Tao*, Aurora Press, Santa Fe; and Chia, M., 1993 *Awaken Healing Light of the Tao*, Healing Tao Books, Huntington.

INDEX